Is There a Father in the House?

A handbook for health and social care professionals

James Torr

Radcliffe Medical Press

Radcliffe Medical Press Ltd
18 Marcham Road
Abingdon
Oxon OX14 1AA
United Kingdom

www.radcliffe-oxford.com
The Radcliffe Medical Press electronic catalogue and online ordering facility.
Direct sales to anywhere in the world.

British Library Cataloguing in Publication Data

A catalogue record for this book is available from the British Library.

ISBN 1 85775 944 3

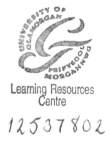

Typeset by Aarontype Ltd, Easton, Bristol
Printed and bound by TJ International Ltd, Padstow, Cornwall

Contents

Preface

Men are in need of positive messages and role models as much as corrective and punitive approaches if their behaviour is to be socially positive. Involved fatherhood is a desirable and socially positive role for men. Negative messages about men's involvement with children do not provide the answer on their own. Men withdraw from involvement with children if their interaction with them is only perceived negatively. Fatherhood then becomes invisible and underestimated.

Services that aim to support fathers' parenting are thinly spread and reactive. Debate focuses on how to recruit fathers to programmes. With nine out of ten fathers now attending the birth of their children, there is a real opportunity to support fathers' involvement with their children. Men are particularly receptive at the birth. The processes before and after the birth also represent an opportunity to support father involvement. Once they are involved, fathers tend to remain so, and involved fathers benefit both women and children.

At present, fathers' needs during this period are overlooked. The emphasis is placed on their role as supporter, but overlooking their needs does not help them to fulfil this role. The role is heavily scripted for mothers and fathers. The emphasis that health professionals put on this role predicates fatherhood as a secondary condition of parenthood and undermines fathers' involvement. It also suggests to mothers that they 'gatekeep' fathers' involvement in the family. Women receive less support as a consequence of this.

Fathers want to support their partners and are also concerned for the health of their babies. Equally, however, they want to be recognised as part of the parenting duo. They do not want to take over maternity services. As a concept, parenthood appeals more than fatherhood. The information needs of fathers are similar to those of mothers. Contradicting stereotypes, fathers want to be involved with their children. Fathers' involvement with their offspring is subject to barriers that undermine their active parenting.

Fathers are given little information either before or after the birth, and virtually none of what they do receive is given to them directly. Giving the father information via the mother burdens the mother and promotes gatekeeping. Hospital environments have few images of involved fathers, and fathers are not always made welcome. The presence of the fathers at the birth is accepted, but this acceptance is undermined by their being ignored afterwards. Mothers become patients and fathers become visitors. Thus health professionals visiting the home overlook the father's needs and involvement.

Men have no common vocabulary of involved parenting, and they underestimate their involvement in their families. This compounds the invisibility of their involvement. Fathers' groups may not be the best means of disseminating information and promoting involvement. Men need information that is aware of masculine perspectives, yet which recognises more than stereotyped interactions with their sons and daughters. Men want information and recognition as parents to be given to them directly.

It is for couples themselves to agree how to share their parenting. The relationship between parents informs campaigns against cot death and the promotion of breastfeeding. Health professionals should recognise relationships and promote dialogue between couples with regard to their joint expectations of father involvement.

James Torr
June 2003

About the author

James Torr is the father of two children, a daughter born in 1995 and a son born in 2001, and thus has recent experience of what are known as maternity services. Prior to undertaking the specific research for this book, he worked on several projects with Fathers Direct, a Home Office funded father support charity, including as senior researcher commissioning articles for a new magazine for practitioners working with fathers, and as a spokesman for the charity in the media and at the Childcare Commission. As well as major funding application drafting he also took part in the foundation of a UK-wide network of practitioners working with fathers and the importing of a US developed training course for professionals and project workers.

Before this, he was a solicitor in a large commercial City firm and became, by choice, a primary carer father in 1995 and subsequently spent three years on the management committee of a registered charity playgroup where he wrote a successful application for National Lottery funding. Additionally, he facilitated what was called its 'mother and toddler group' (a name later changed to 'parent and toddler group'). The author is presently chair of the City of London Parents Group which works with the local authority and a cross-boundary health project to secure improved services for families and children in the various resident communities of the City.

Prologue

A father at home

By 1993, my partner and I had reached the point in our relationship and our careers where our thoughts were turning more and more towards starting a family. During this period, looking back over my own upbringing in what became a time of personal turmoil, I felt strongly motivated to 'be there' for my own child and determined to be a present and caring parent. I felt as sure about this as I felt boxed in by expectations about my career. To my confusion, I still held some of these.

Despite this, I was essentially unhappy with many aspects of my career as a City solicitor, working on large and stressful transactions about buildings I never saw for anonymous corporate clients whose apparatchiks I barely ever met. The partners in the firm at the time were not around much to help you out. I was well paid, but I was not satisfied. However, my partner was settled and secure in her career as a teacher.

We conceived our first child in 1995, having agreed, in one of the shortest conversations we have ever had, that I would look after our newborn child at home.

An involved dad in public

Although I was convinced of the value of our decision as far as our new family was concerned, I was less certain how this decision would go down publicly. This uncertainty was reflected and increased by the mixed reaction that our decision caused within our families of origin. I felt this particularly in the context of the career expectations that both families had for me, which implicated me both as a man and as a father.

According to these expectations, it seemed broadly acceptable for a mother to work, but it was not so acceptable for a father to look after the children. On the other hand, there was something of an understanding that it was desirable that one parent should stay at home to look after the children, at least in the early years. So my decision to do this as a father caused both positive and negative reactions within our families. Overall, however, the tenor of these reactions had the character of bemused and slightly stunned disbelief. There were no angry confrontations where my decision was explicitly at issue, although there have been others where it was all but named. However, informing the many reactions was the fundamental belief that parenting was not a 'proper job', irrespective of the scorn that might be heaped upon delinquent children brought up by neglectful parents.

So men had jobs and women looked after children. As it was broadly acceptable for women to work, perhaps it would be all the more appropriate if this job should be in the compromise position of looking after children in one form or another. Yet the actual functions of parenting and childcare were held in near contempt, despite their perceived benefit to young children. What did this say about society's attitude to women? And what did it say about how it values children, regardless of the tidal waves of sentiment concerning them that have been so prevalent in recent years? Thus, although I was nominally encountering many of these issues because of my decision to become an engaged father at home, it appeared that I had inadvertently exposed some uncomfortable underlying attitudes about parenting, children and childcare as a whole.

However, at this level these were private concerns that I thought bore only upon us and our families. Moreover, there was nothing particularly uncommon about these attitudes, which seemed to be shared in many quarters.

Becoming a dad at home, though, soon enough had a public dimension. It is impossible to spend all day every day indoors, even if one wants to. At the very minimum you have to go out to buy food and nappies. Most parents have at least one supermarket experience with their young children that stays in their mind. One such encounter occurred when my daughter was coming to the boil just as the checkout queue almost came to a halt. Eventually we reached the checkout worker, who kindly said 'Poor little girl, where's your mummy?'.

At the level of our local community, when the time came to begin to introduce our child to other children, I encountered barriers to making contacts with other parents. Obviously the difference in sex was the main one. Despite the fact that it is very easy for the engaged father to slip into the habit of describing them as 'other mothers', mothers nonetheless tend to react to what they see – that is, a man, even though he is doing the same job. Perhaps there is something to note here for those men who are afraid of childcare because it will be perceived to compromise their masculinity. There is less reason to be anxious about this than might be thought, for the fact that you are a man will probably not be overlooked for a single moment.

However, not all full-time mothers want to join the gang, and cliques form among groups of men as well. It is not always the case that you want to join them. It makes sense to remind yourself that it takes time to be accepted by any group of people, and not to attribute the initial isolation to gender.

Once it is perceived that you share the same concerns about your child's development as anyone else and this is where your focus lies, acceptance begins. This is the first hurdle. You can then succeed in arranging for your child to be able to play in the park after nursery or school with some of his or her peers.

The second hurdle is moving these connections into the private sphere, and making new ones beyond the aegis of school, nursery or drop-in. Here there are issues that require a sensitive and tactical approach. In the case of some parents whom you meet, these issues will remain insurmountable and you will have to accept this and make friends for your child elsewhere.

The main issue is how you invite a mother into your home, when both of your partners are at work, without the invitation looking suspicious to others. If you ask the wrong mother at the wrong time, before you know it you can find yourself in a kind of hall of mirrors of erroneous perceptions and assumptions.

Get it badly wrong, and the first assumption she might make in response to your suggesting that her child could come home to tea with yours is that you are making a pass at her. In the unskilled early months of this phase of your child's development, this will be one of those necessary learning experiences. However, you have not entered the hall of mirrors this time – you have just been refused entry at the door. This will probably happen if not enough time has been spent in making the initial acquaintance and showing that 'where you are at' is not about the mother concerned except in so far as she is the parent of a similarly-aged child to your own who could potentially spend some time with your child as a friend.

You enter the hall of mirrors when you have correctly identified and made acquaintance with one like-minded person, but a person who focuses on extraneous anxieties associated with other peoples' perceived opinions. Certainly you are judged not to be making a pass at her yourself – you have given out the right messages here – but she still might think about your partner or wife. Is your partner or wife accepting of this proposal? If she appears to be that accepting of it, then perhaps she might conclude that there is actually something untoward going on after all. Then she might think of her own partner or husband. Would he be happy about her being in another man's home or him being in their home escorted only by a couple of very young children? She might not think this is an issue, but it is important to be aware that her partner will probably regard it as such. If it is not one of these scenarios, it might just be a case of non-specific anxiety about how it appears to spend time in the company of another man and what it looks like for that guy to suggest it, even if you are getting the message that the woman concerned does not actually think that your personal motives are suspect.

It is possible over time to meet like-minded people – this is rewarding both for you and for your children – or situations can be contrived by measures such as asking two mothers and their children home at the same time, but this kind of success tends to be achieved by swimming somewhat against the tide. Thus moving connections into the private sphere requires long-term development. In the short term it is easier to make connections with the parents of other children in a public or shared space, such as a nursery or drop-in. It can also be easier to get along with paid carers, for whom the idea of a father being involved often seems to be less of an issue, as perhaps they are only contingent members of the club themselves.

Facilitating a parent and toddler group: issues for men in childcare

In my community this group was called the 'mother and toddler group'. Nonetheless, the leader of the nearby playgroup met me a few times, as she also met my partner, and each time she warmly insisted that I was welcome to come. Before long the playgroup was going to close unless someone volunteered to keep it going by opening it up and collecting the small admission fee. It became an important resource for me, and I was beginning to feel that I had something to prove.

I felt in a similar position to those women who were among the first wave to go out to work in the 1960s and 1970s, but in my case what was being judged was not my performance at work, but my performance as a parent. I felt, as was so often experienced by those women going into the office for the first time, that I had to reach a higher standard of performance in order to justify doing the job at all.

In a sense my 'running' of the group – which actually meant getting there whatever the weather or however reluctant I felt before opening time, collecting the admission fee and names of visitors, making the tea, doing the washing up, leading the music session at the end, tidying up after everyone had left and organising the Christmas party – was the price of my admission to it. I felt that my presence could not be challenged if I undertook all of these tasks on behalf of the people who used the drop-in. However, as time went on, the group became established and people volunteered to help out.

I am still proud of the contribution that I made. Later, at a conference workshop, I remarked that I had 'run' a toddler group (this somehow being relevant to the topic under discussion). This provoked the response, in a written letter of complaint that followed, that as a man I had obviously enjoyed feeling 'in charge' of a group of women. The inference was that this was why I had sought to take part in the way I did. However, I felt that – if anything – the truth was that the women had actually determined the role I played in the group, and that it was their expectations that led to it. Meeting those expectations was, for me, the price of my admission. I don't think it was me who was in charge.

What is interesting here is that in primary schools and other childcare environments where men and women work together with children, the men (who are always in a minority) are often allotted technical or management roles (e.g. treasurer) by a kind of invisible process that leads them away from front-line contact with the children. Typically in a primary school, for example, the one male teacher will be the Head. Alternatively, they may be given 'male' tasks such as DIY. Nonetheless, however even-handed this process may be between the men and women who take part in it, the charge is often made (as it was in my case) that even when they are in a minority it is the men's instinct to 'take over' the management of the environment in which they find themselves. Often the higher salaries that they earn in managerial roles are a source of some of this resentment. Again, however, I do not think that this process of moving the men 'upstairs' or into other technical roles and away from front-line contact with children is determined solely by men's expectations.

So although I encountered many of these issues because of my decision to become an engaged father at home, I was becoming aware of some uncomfortable underlying attitudes in society about parenting, children and childcare as a whole that being a full-time father only exposed afresh.

I was aware that many mothers also felt pressure to return to work simply because of the low value attached to parenting in general – whether by mothers or by fathers. This was highlighted by the Government drive to get single parents (at that time, as now, almost exclusively described as 'single mothers') off benefits and into work in a campaign that seemed to convey that stay-at-home parenting was lazy, valueless and undertaken only by economic losers.

Thus all parents were being judged critically in a culture of blame that held them responsible both for their acts and for the acts of their children, without valuing the remedy of active and present parenting. Campaigns against working motherhood in some popular newspapers, which cited allegedly adverse outcomes for children, appeared to have as their main goal not so much benefiting children as a too late reactionary focus against women's complete participation in the economy and society. (The latter is something to which full-time parents have incomplete access, as attested to by the derision rightly heaped on Mrs Thatcher's opinion that there is no such thing as society, only families.) The proof of this reactionary focus is that these same newspapers never advocate more engaged fatherhood to fill the supposed gap in these children's lives that has been left by their mothers going out to work. As the crime statistics have increased, particularly because of theft of mobile phones, youth offending has become more prominent in people's consciousness as well as on the streets. However, more recently it has been found that supporting parents in challenging circumstances with parenting classes has reduced youth offending, demonstrating the value of active parenting.

Fathers, on the other hand, at the end of the Thatcher/Major period were coming under fire for failing to meet their responsibilities towards their children when the relationship with the mother broke down. The Child Support Agency was formed to make them indemnify the taxpayer from welfare payments to support their children. The father's responsibilities and the nature of his support were perceived in exclusively financial terms. As with the emphasis in the popular press and media on the value of traditional stay-at-home motherhood, coverage of fatherhood rested on traditional values associated in the father's case with the model of father as breadwinner. Although to this day the courts nearly always award custody of the children to the mother, whatever the father's wishes or relationship with his children and irrespective of the comparative history of their parenting, this becomes translated as the father 'leaving his children', thus reinforcing stereotypes of irresponsibility and fecklessness.

However, at the beginning of the Blair Government the adverse focus on men and fathers moved up a gear. Many of the new Labour women MPs had an interest in family matters, but one that centred on women and children. At the major biannual family services conference, Parent Child 2000, held in London, the conference was opened by a Government minister who confined her remarks to mothers for the whole of her opening speech. Men in general and fathers in particular came in for some terrible news coverage during this period of government. A lot of attention was being paid to the problems that both men and fathers were causing and seemed to be causing – most often in very-broad-brush depictions – in society and in the home. Television and advertising campaigns against domestic violence and child abuse featured men and fathers in centre frame. It was the peak era – or the low point – of the lads' mags and 'Men behaving badly', and it seemed that men were acting out the roles they were given – even if these were destructive.

The criticism of men and fathers presented many problems, some of them all too real. However, initially there seemed to be an unwillingness to offer up solutions other than blanket condemnation (no solution at all in itself, but comfortably situated on the moral high ground). Few, if any, alternative behaviours and positive identities for men seemed to be acknowledged or on offer – least of all from those offering the criticism. On the contrary, there seemed to be a wish to prove, when Beatrix Campbell and others asserted that 'Men are the Problem', that it was not problematic behaviour by men that was at issue, but rather the men themselves. The absence of constructive solutions seemed near total, even willed. Prejudicial statements were made about men and fathers which if applied to an ethnic group would be an offence under the Public Order Acts as an incitement to racial hatred. Misogyny was well defined, but it was open season on men and fathers.

Children were defined as absolutely good. Poor parenting was to blame for all problematic behaviour by children. If society made and enjoyed watching films that featured heads being cut off, sexual violence and a body count in double figures, it was parents' fault if children watched these films or absorbed their values. Above all, when children were being defined as the only remaining absolute good in society, it amounted to offensive moral relativism to point out that only a tiny minority of men harm them. It was equally offensive moral relativism to point out, as UNESCO did, that the UK has the lowest child mortality rates from accident and abuse apart from Sweden in a survey of 40 countries in the developed world in a report that criticised 'high-profile media treatment of selected cases, and more generalized warnings from public organisations that have to compete for public attention and public funds'.[1]

The offensiveness of these qualifying factors also appears to lie in part in the unresolved anxieties about children that mitigate against their wished-for iconic status of being an absolute good in an uncertain world. In my local community, skateboarding children are viewed with an enmity and hostility that far exceeds any real threat which some might argue they pose. It is perhaps fears and anxieties such as these which demonstrate that much of the sentimental conceptualisation of children seems to contain little evidence of their being valued by society in their complexity, as they actually are. On the contrary, many of the prevailing sentimental views about children appear to be sourced in an idealised, hoped-for vision, rather than in how they are often experienced, by people who bring their own expectations about children with them. What these expectations may in fact reveal is a real hostility towards the way children can actually present themselves. This hostility was notably revealed by the Jamie Bulger case, which exposed on the same coin the sentimentalising of children on the one face and profound fears on the reverse face that some children, far from satisfying such a need to be inherently good, might on the contrary pose the threat of being inherently evil. These fears were exploited in a Conservative Party election broadcast in 2001, for example, which featured feral truants let loose by negligent and poorly managed teachers to wreak havoc on the streets. When children fail to satisfy the need to be 'an absolute good', they can be treated with a vindictiveness which goes way beyond any kind of proportionate response to any offence they may commit.

Above all, in these sensitised and unresolved parallel debates about men and children, men having contact with children was now considered to be inherently and indeed doubly problematic. Paedophiles competed with the Internet as the filler story on a slow news day, and made headlines every other day as well. Most sensational of all were the growing number of stories about paedophiles conspiring together on the Internet. However, the mud about men and children – including fathers and their own children – was beginning to stick. Once an idea has been received, it becomes timelessly repeated, told and retold like a myth. The retelling even occurs when the storyteller and the listener may both doubt the objective truth of the idea. The truth is less important than meeting the needs of the teller and listener in the familiarity of the tale, and the comfort of the repetition in founding a collective reference point.

Thus when the National Society for the Prevention of Cruelty to Children (NSPCC) conducted one of the largest surveys on child abuse in the UK[2] and found that fathers were minority perpetrators in cases of both sexual and physical abuse of children, it went largely unreported in relative terms.[3] Indeed, writing in the *Guardian* at the time, Dea Birkett took issue with these findings that challenged a group belief. Writing about sexual abuse, she said 'Only 14% of this abuse was said to be carried out by the person we would most readily point a finger at – the father. ... It is a phenomenal claim.'[4]

In Birkett's canon it is not the truth that counts, but what 'we' believe to be the truth. Challenging a collective reference point becomes a challenge to the collective. But who is this 'we' that Birkett writes for? Is it meant to include fathers themselves? And what are they then to do with the knowledge that 'we' believe them to be culpable, irrespective of the facts? It is almost as if it is an insult on their part against the collective if they behave in ways that the collective has not sanctioned by recognition, if they do *not* abuse their children. In any case, whatever Birkett's view and whether the statistics are right or wrong, the last way to lead men out of problem behaviours is to tell them that it is determined by society's belief that they will inevitably display those behaviours.

Thus I began to discover that parenting as a whole was undervalued, that economic values prevailed, and that the legitimacy of men having contact with children — even their own — was at issue. It is not as if most men were unaware of or unaffected by this. Stories about the culture of long working hours also began to increase at this time. Uncertain of their value and position in the home, and influenced by the exclusive endorsement of the economic values pertaining to them as breadwinners, notably by the Child Support Agency, men started to spend even longer in the office. Then came the charge, in subsequent news items and from Jack Straw, the Home Secretary at the time, that men were neglecting their children and spending too little time with them. Again it was as if men's expectations alone had determined this development — just as men being subject to criticism for 'taking over' management jobs that led them away from front-line work with children in childcare settings was posited as a development driven exclusively by men's expectations.

I was asked to join the committee of the community playgroup that my daughter moved on to. One reason given for this was that apart from having helped at the toddler drop-in as a father, I could provide a 'needed' male perspective. At that time there were no fathers on a large committee made up only of parents. I did not see it as necessarily ironic that, as a father, I joined it as one of the small minority of full-time parents who gave their time to it. I thought it more symbolic of a modern society where individuals and families could make their own socially responsible choices without having to play roles and observe expectations in a social theatre for which the scripts were written in the 1950s or even earlier.

Therefore I thought it anomalous that my fellow committee members (high-powered lawyers and businesspeople, as was plainly evident in our meetings) seemed to slip back into cooking and baking roles when organising events. I felt that I recognised in this aspects of my own behaviour when, in the more self-conscious early days, I would let my wife push our child's pram. It seemed that the socially conservative scripts of the 1950s still held power over both men and women, particularly where the context was suggestive of distinct roles that each should play. On bonfire night in November, the women made the soup and the men lit the fireworks.

The issue of the power of suggestion (as in the role expectations described above) acting both positively and negatively on men and women and their relationships is one of the principal themes of this book. This power of suggestion is stronger in some contexts than in others, but perhaps no more so than in maternity services — environments where many new parents, forming their first impressions, are either anxious about the birth and their newborn, trusting of health professionals, keen to do the right thing, or all of these.

The structural forces that drive gender role differentiation include the power of suggestion in these environments, but wider forces in society (such as those touched upon and illustrated above) also bring considerable pressure to bear upon individuals, and should also be borne in mind when professionals are reflecting on more specific issues of practice. As Daniel and Taylor remark:

> Theories of oppression warn us, therefore, that we cannot work in an anti-sexist way without taking account of structural forces. The failure to examine these forces and how they impact on the individual explains why simple exhortations to men to be more involved have minimal effect and, of course, why simple exhortations to practitioners to engage with fathers have minimal effect. Structural forces affect us all, and it is not easy for an individual to adopt gender role behaviour usually associated with the opposite sex.[5]

Thus mother–child-centred models of caring which overlook the presence of the father in a family with an expected or a newborn child can themselves become part of these structural forces. Such models, which do not bring the father into the process, suggest to the mother that allowing the father to become involved may not be consistent with her assigned gender role, which is fulfilled by being the complete parent on her own. Equally, they suggest to the father that it runs counter to his gender role to become involved and be an active partner in parenting.

At the playgroup committee, I was so keen to fit in that in reality my being a father had relatively little impact. Despite the fact of my being a father having been given as one reason for my joining the committee, issues relevant to exploring fathers' needs and perspectives were never raised or explored. Moreover, I found it difficult for one father to speak for all of them. Phrases like 'here we are, a group of mothers' were regularly used in meetings. Or 'James, you're running a mothers-and-toddlers group – how are things going there?'. One or two might wince and look at me – I spent a lot of time fundraising for the playgroup.

Nonetheless, I suggested that the name of the drop-in group for the toddlers should be changed to the 'parents, carers and toddlers group', to make it more accessible to fathers and the other carers who brought children to attend the group. To add weight to my suggestion that the name 'mothers and toddlers group' be changed, I reminded the committee that the two people who had worked at the group over the previous year had been a father and a grandmother. The change was rejected, but the name 'parents and toddlers group' was accepted instead. It is possible that 'carers' was too modern-sounding a term, but there was something of a sense that the other parents on the committee did not want to cede any more of their stake in a group that paid carers often attended in practice.

Although the change was made to the name on the letterhead, it has not been generally accepted in practice. It remains an issue that has not been fully resolved and which has caused some resentment. On site, the old name of 'mothers and toddlers' is used by the staff. The suggestion was later made to me by a new committee member that the new name was designed to include 'anyone but mothers'.

After a while, the idea of hiring a male childcare worker for the playgroup was briefly discussed by the committee. A female member of staff had previously asked mothers bringing their children to the playgroup what they thought about this. Because of fears of child abuse which had been expressed, the idea was not taken forward. I felt that I was in no position to challenge these fears – there was a lot of coverage of child abuse by the media, and I was the one man on a committee of ten members. I did not want to create controversy, and instead I sought to show that a man could work constructively as a team member. It was impossible to argue that if a man was hired, nothing bad would happen. Yet the fact that it was equally impossible to argue that if a woman was hired nothing bad would happen was a completely academic consideration and would not have counted at all. No systems for providing reassurance, such as procedures for escorting children to the lavatory, were considered either before or after the soundings were made. There was an uncomfortable atmosphere while the soundings were being reported by the member of staff, and her recommendation not to proceed was accepted without argument. No fathers or other men had been asked for their views during the initial soundings.

I thought back to the strange reaction shown by the health visitor when she first came to our home and was told that I was going to be the primary carer. Her response was to reassure me that it was 'OK' for me to show affection towards our daughter.

There did not seem to be any focus on how fathers, or men working with children, could get it right or be supported. I thought I was doing a good (or at least conscientious) job. However, I was a stay-at-home father, and my decision was therefore relatively unusual. It seemed to offer no wider lessons. I had no idea how many men were doing the same thing as me, but I guessed it was a relatively small number. There was little to be gleaned from the articles by stay-at-home fathers that occasionally cropped up as interesting diversions in the lifestyle pages in the press. At the time, too, references to single parents nearly always excluded single fathers as a matter of definition.

Around this time, at the birthday party of a friend's daughter, I met a handful of other fathers, all of whom were working fathers. I was struck by how caring and attentive they all were. Like some others before, they expressed regret that they could not spend as much time with their children as I could with mine. I felt a connection with these men who cared for their children.

I had not heard anything about great dads like these in the media, but it did not seem to me they could be as uncommon as all that. Rather, it seemed that if 'bad dads' were the problem, the attitudes and commitment of caring fathers such as these were the solution. And these were working fathers, who had a majority stake among fathers.

I began to think that if men as a whole were being defined as the problem because of their behaviour, was not attentive and involved parenting by these men a good way of being a man? But how could fathers feel encouraged with all of the focus on abusive men by the media?

It seemed to me that this focus acted to prevent men from caring for children, just as so many were being criticised for failing to do so. It seemed to me also that little account was being taken of the barriers which prevented men looking after children (of the kind I felt I had observed myself when it came to the question of hiring a male childcare worker).

In that instance, I felt that the essentially socially conservative values of my community had operated as a barrier against men looking after children, which had been raised even higher by an admixture of ostensibly progressive, ideologically founded stereotypes about the abusiveness of men. It seemed that as socially conservative prescriptions about the distinctiveness of gender roles were being generally challenged in many areas, in the field of childcare ideologically founded stereotypes about abusive men were paradoxically undermining men's role in childcare. Nominally progressive views were being used to socially conservative ends. It struck me most that although men were often the subject of criticism for failing to look after children, among all the parents who were actively involved in deciding against hiring a male childcare worker, none of them had been a father.

I felt that it was also something of an irony that the working parents on the committee had benefited directly or indirectly from equal opportunities legislation which had, quite rightly, lowered many of the barriers that they faced in reaching the top of their professions. Yet the decision that was reached about hiring a male childcare worker amounted to the exclusion from employment of one gender by another that none of them would have found acceptable in their professional lives.

I also felt that there was a resistance to the idea of men looking after children that was not completely explained by fears about child abuse. Indeed, it seemed to me to be possible that many of these fears were an expression of that resistance. There seemed to be a reluctance to let men get involved in the business of child-care. But neither was it clear to me that this reluctance necessarily stopped at the door of the family home, or that it only involved men other than the father looking after the children, despite all of the surveys one heard about where fathers were being criticised for not taking part in childcare.

It appeared that fathers were receiving very mixed messages about the value of their involvement with children and the terms of that involvement. Men's confidence in that value was also, and remains, undermined by the absence of a 'way forward' for fatherhood when male nurturing is perceived to be problematic as a change of emphasis from the traditional model of fatherhood. Developments in the modern economy tended to undermine their traditional role. Developments in modern society worked as much against them exercising a more caring function as they did to encourage them. These developments coalesced around a growing debate as to whether fathers were in fact necessary at all, either socially or ultimately in biological terms. But how were fathers to perform well in either a traditional or a modern capacity when the question of whether they were needed at all was so often at issue? It seemed easier to discount their value as a whole than to decide what was the nature of the value they could bring to children and families, and then to acknowledge that value.

Many fathers were apparently not performing well. This fuelled the debate about their value in what I saw as a self-fulfilling cycle of negative expectations and outcomes. An essentially prejudiced view of men was not reaping positive rewards, but whenever it was put to any kind of test, it tended to seek its own justification. However, rather than the focus remaining on the fathers themselves in this way, I felt that this negative dynamic in the debate made it urgently important to address structural forces like those exerted by the debate itself that bore upon fathers and men externally and acted adversely on their involvement with their families and society. Once these issues had been addressed, it would be possible to review afresh the 'positives' that fathers and men themselves could bring to balance the equation within a framework of partnership and co-operation. Positive expectations, when agreed upon between men and women, could then lead to positive outcomes.

Such agreement must of necessity be founded upon open dialogue between the parties to the debate. It must involve all parties admitting the shortcomings of their actions and attitudes, and simultaneous positive action from both parties working in partnership to remedy specific identified problems. In this context, it is important to acknowledge that men's behaviour can cause many problems for families and society. But that said, it is important to move the debate on beyond the identification of problems, and to attempt to seek solutions that both men and women can bring to a resolution of the debate that will provide a framework of positive expectation, which can lead to the growth of positive outcomes. The problems posed by antisocial behaviour by men are therefore not dwelt on at length in this book. This is because these issues have been examined in depth elsewhere and in many respects are not a matter of contention. However, they have also not been dwelt on at length because the search for solutions must envisage other, positive behaviours and the means of bringing them about. This is equally why the harm that is done to children by women (where sometimes in such cases it is the women who are unsupported by the men, and men are also failing to bring positives to the situation) is not addressed in this book, apart from considering how men can better support women. The search for solutions and positive behaviours includes acknowledging existing positive behaviour by men in a reverse of the negative expectation–negative outcome dynamic. It is essential, and entirely rational, to incorporate this acknowledgement into the debate without fearing that the existence of negative behaviour by men is being challenged by it. This is the sense in which the debate has to expand and move on.

It is suggested that within the construction of a framework of agreement and partnership that can bring about such positive outcomes, women can help to bring as much to the equation as men. Women can support men in the interests of children just as in those situations referred to above where men can support women in the interests of children. This does not imply the reverse perspective – that women are responsible for or 'ask for' negative behaviour by men. Again the search for solutions has to move beyond an introverted debate of this kind that seeks primarily to lay blame rather than to remedy problems. So where it is suggested that men or women consider new courses of action, it is moreover to imply that the human spirit has the potential to bring out positive behaviours from others that it would be absurd to imply reflected adversely on that spirit.

Working with a charity that supports fathers

I heard of a new charity that had produced a guide to fatherhood for new dads. I had noticed it because it was the first good-news story about dads in the press for a long time. The charity was organising a conference about developing effective services for fathers to support their parenting. These services were essential if men were getting it as wrong as they were supposed to be doing, but they were – and still are – very thin on the ground.

I shared some thoughts and ideas with the charity, and started working with it part-time, juggling work with my daughter's school hours and the occasional begged, borrowed or stolen hour of childcare. Without my partner's involvement, despite the constraints of her full-time job, little of this would have been possible.

James Torr
June 2003

References

1   United Nations (International) Children's (Emergency) Fund (UNICEF) (2001) *A League Table of Child Deaths by Injury in Rich Nations*. Innocenti Report Card No. 2. UNICEF Innocenti Research Centre, Florence, pp. 20–1.
2   National Society for the Prevention of Cruelty to Children (NSPCC) (2000) *Child Maltreatment in the UK: a study of the prevalence of child abuse and neglect*. NSPCC, London.
3   Child abuse 'myths' shattered; *BBC News Online*, 20 November 2000.
4   Birkett D (2000) Why little boys are not sex offenders. *Guardian*. **21 November**.
5   Daniel B and Taylor J (2001) *Engaging with Fathers: practice issues for health and social care*. Jessica Kingsley Publishers, London, p. 217.

CHAPTER 1

Introduction

The work of a charity supporting fathers: where do you start?

- The focus is not on 'men's rights'. The work focuses on helping all fathers, resident and non-resident, with their involvement with their children. Priority is not given to men going through the process of divorce or lone or primary carer fathers specifically.

Fathers Direct seeks to promote close and positive relationships between men and their children. It provides information for fathers through its website www.fathers direct.com, and *The Bounty Guide to Fatherhood*, which is distributed free in the Bounty Mother-To-Be pack to 650 000 families a year.

It also aims to lower barriers to involved fatherhood by supporting the development of family services that are accessible to fathers, and it advocates more flexible working practices for parents. It seeks to challenge gender stereotypes that limit both men and women and reduce the quality of parenting for children. More generally, it seeks to highlight good fathering and create a culture that is supportive of dads raising children by interventions in the media.

The first *FatherWork* magazine for practitioners working with fathers, for which I was senior researcher, was published in May 2001.

Listening to fathers calling for help

- Men want to be involved parents.
- Barriers exist which inhibit men's parenting.
- These barriers lie both within men and within society.
- For example, men's working hours in the UK are the longest in Europe.
- Few services exist either to assist men in overcoming these barriers or to support their parenting.

The principal working assumption was that men wish and have the potential to be involved parents, that this involvement is beneficial to them and to the women and children in their lives, and that at times it can be appropriate to help to unlock that potential. This assumption was supported by the view that where a father needed support with his parenting, this might be as much because of factors external to him operating against his involvement as it might be due to factors within his control. Sometimes it is difficult to distinguish between these factors, as men can adopt external factors, such as a generalised societal belief that children are better cared for by their mothers.

The starting assumption was not that men are necessarily dangerous and that women and children therefore always need protection from them, nor was it that they have no wish to be active parents. Assumptions such as these can in fact be seen as examples of the barriers that inhibit active parenting by men and tend to operate against positive outcomes from men's interaction with women and children. Such barriers are manifestations of the 'structural forces' identified by Daniel and Taylor that can operate on fathers and act against their involvement with their children. In the examples given here, the first assumption leads to a belief that men and children should be kept apart because of the risks to children (this includes male childcare workers), and the second assumption contributes to a belief that when they are present, necessarily uninterested fathers bring no value to their children. This in turn leads to the view that their parenting is not worth supporting or valuing, in what becomes a downward spiral of expectations and outcomes.

The aim in practice was – in contrast to the above assumptions – to start from a fundamentally positive view of men and fathers and to address each barrier to involved fatherhood in turn, thereby seeking a means of lowering each of them.

As well as researching for the *FatherWork* practitioners' magazine and intervening in media debates, I manned the office helpline that takes calls from professionals and fathers. I also helped to organise training for professionals working with fathers, with seminars by experienced trainers from the USA. It was clear that there was a great need for services to support fathers' parenting which was not being met.

Perhaps the most powerful experience attesting to men's capacity to love and care for their children comes not from the studies which support the contention that they want to be involved parents or future parents, but from hearing fathers themselves talking about their experience of fatherhood. As part of the professional training workshops and seminars for those working with fathers or newly embarking on family support projects which include fathers, the common formula is to interview a panel. The fathers on the panel talk about their experience of any support which they have been offered, so that the professionals in the audience can seek to replicate the positive aspects and avoid the negative ones. The courage and spirit of the men I have heard speaking out on such panels about their love for their children – what is for them a deeply personal matter – is profoundly affecting.

Many fathers rang the helpline because they were desperate and could find no services to help them, or had no idea of where to go locally. They had often never been engaged with by any agency, so had no idea where to turn. They called the office because they had heard of us in the media. Often just knowing that there were people out there supporting them seemed to be of value.

This in itself seemed to offer a lesson. Often a relatively small amount of support, delivered at the right time in the right way, can appear to have as beneficial an effect as cost-heavy structured interventions. Sometimes too much support, or support delivered in a ham-fisted manner, can threaten a man's sense of being perceived to be in command of himself.

For example, in my own case my partner and I were interviewed by a paedia-trician after the birth of our first child. When he asked what it was I did, and I told him that I was going to stay at home and look after my daughter, he looked at his notes and said, while he was writing, 'I'm putting down FTF – that's the short-hand I always use for full-time father'. He did not blink an eye or say any more – nor did he need to. My confidence in what I was doing was bolstered enough without my ever getting the feeling that I was being talked down to.

Another crucial point relating to the professional's practice in this example is that as the father I was actually interviewed and asked the question in the first place. This does not always happen, even when the father is resident within the family home and easily accessible. In my own case, in 2001 after the birth of our second child no such question was put to me by the health visitor, who conducted the whole interview on the assumption that I would be back at work and out of the home in a couple of weeks. I had opened the door to her while I was holding our child. When the health visitor left, my partner was holding him.

My experience in the latter instance was one of marginalisation. This also occurred when the visiting midwives attended. I had been at the birth, seen the blood, cut the umbilical cord and nursed and fed my partner through exhaustion and fever for three days after she was discharged from hospital. On the first visit to our home there was a sense of expectation from the visiting professional that I would leave the room. On this visit, as with the rest, no questions or points were addressed to me, but I was specifically thanked for changing a nappy. It is a point made later in this book that models of practice such as these, that marginalise fathers, have an adverse impact on involvement by all fathers (be they at home, or working part-time or full-time) and thus tend to impose all of the burdens of parenting on the mother. Such models of practice tend to act as one of the barriers to men's involvement with their children that it was the charity's objective to address and to attempt to lower.

Listening to the experiences of other fathers, perhaps the most distressing call I took at the office was from a recently widowed father. He was struggling with the grief of bereavement at the same time as he was experiencing isolation as a single male parent. Not one friend had come round to play with his daughter in six months, and he felt excluded and marginalised by the mothers who were reluctant to let their daughters go to his house. This made him feel a failure as a carer. Until recently, single parenthood has been an issue considered only to affect women, but one in ten single parents is a father. There are also at least 100 000 stay-at-home carer-fathers,[1] but this figure is probably significantly under-reported, as many men probably cite their former occupations in surveys.

Many fathers are struggling to be both active parents and valued employees. Fathers in the UK work the longest hours in Europe, but employers are often reluctant to acknowledge that men as well as women can be committed parents. Discrimination against parents in the workplace acts as a barrier against fathers as well as mothers, yet with the exception of parental and paternal leave, there is no legislation designed to protect fathers (although it can haphazardly operate to this effect on occasion). The Gingerbread Report on lone fathers, for example, found that they can experience a '"glass ceiling" effect similar to that associated with women workers.'[2]

When the pay gap between men and women is analysed, the difference is often most marked with regard to part-time work. However, these calculations ignore the fact that part-time work is seldom available to men, or made available if it is requested. Fathers called who were encountering another type of barrier to their parenting, namely when their careers were in difficulty because they had requested a variation in their working hours in order to accommodate their family commitments. Pay calculations based on those few senior executives with a portfolio of part-time directorships and the bargaining power to determine their work-life balance should not give the impression that part-time work is something which is only structured against women's participation in the economy. It is also structured against men's involvement with their families, because it is so rarely available to them. Some would go on to argue that if part-time work were made more widely available to men, pay rates would rise on the basis that all work by women is undervalued.

There were and still are many issues to address. Work-life balance, attitudes to gender roles (including the father's traditional role as breadwinner), fears about child abuse, and health professionals' models of practice are just some of the issues that are all competing for time, attention and resources. Supporting fathers in dealing with all of these issues is an enormous task. However, the issue that is currently receiving attention, particularly in the family support sector, is a more primary one. It concerns how to reach fathers on an individual rather than a policy level, how to bring them in to attend support programmes, and how best to help and support their parenting effectively by other means. Some aspects of the challenges here have already been raised (e.g. how to do this without threatening an individual's sense of being perceived to be in command of himself). These issues are the subject of the practice sections of this book, but perhaps the most significant opportunity to reach fathers arises around the time of the birth of their children.

The significance of the birth for fathers and family support services

- There is an overall lack of services to support fathers' parenting.
- Services have difficulty in accessing fathers.
- Nine out of ten fathers attend the birth of their children.
- Fathers are particularly receptive at this time.
- An opportunity therefore arises to access fathers before problems arise, and to bond men positively to their children, partnerships and society.
- Men want recognition as parents, but they do not wish to take over maternity services. Their main concerns are for the health of their partner and babies.
- The attitudes of workers about men and fathers can determine whether fathers are given this recognition.
- Providing fathers with the information that they need helps to give them recognition as parents, which improves the quality of their parenting.
- Fathers' information needs are similar to those of mothers, but an awareness of masculine perspectives may be important.

The National Family and Parenting Institute (NFPI) recently conducted a survey of family support services which identified 'very few services specifically targeted at minority ethnic groups and fathers.'[3] It found that fathers were an 'excluded group'.

Some new projects, particularly those associated with local Sure Start initiatives, as well as the NFPI itself, are beginning to address the imbalance and are looking at how to access fathers, or make existing services that support parents more accessible to them. Often this involves lengthy and persistent outreach and community development work with heavy time resource expenditure in bringing fathers to attend programmes. On the other hand, some projects are over-used as referral options by 'mainstream' parent support services that are unused to dealing with fathers.

However, if support services are asking how their projects can access fathers to sustain them as parents, and which fathers to support most cost-effectively, a service that is currently proactively sought out by nine out of ten fathers must be regarded as a significant opportunity. With nine out of ten fathers attending the birth of their children, there in fact seems to be an opportunity going begging.

Overstretched maternity services may not welcome being cast as a family support service, but this is wholly consistent with preventive principles, to which some do subscribe at the moment. This has been put into practice, for example, in hospitals where new mothers are screened by midwives for signs of abuse by their partners.

Of the few projects that currently exist to support fathers' parenting, most if not all aim to repair relationships that are already damaged or in some kind of difficulty. A preventive approach must therefore be argued for according to the conclusions of a recent UK study, which found that 'early father involvement with a child is associated with continuing involvement with that child throughout childhood and adolescence.'[4] This report found that involved fatherhood is associated with a range of beneficial outcomes for children. A 'preventive' approach taken here would therefore bring additional positive benefits. Some of those benefits will be examined in greater detail in the section below on the value to children of involved fathers (see p. 39).

The evidence that is particularly compelling in the context of early father involvement concerns the significance of the birth for fathers, and the opportunity that this affords to assist their active and involved parenting. However, it also appears that bringing fathers into the process is achievable within current procedures. Fathers do not want to take over. Their principal concerns focus on the health of their unborn and newborn children and that of their partners. But equally they do not want to be marginalised, and they seek recognition as one half of the parenting duo.

This recognition, it is argued below, does not call for a whole new expertise in the information that parents need in order to include fathers. Studies show that their information needs are largely the same as those of mothers. What may be required is some adaptation in information delivery to meet their needs that easily justifies the marginal expenditure required. The fact that fathers are particularly receptive at the time of the birth is a further argument for resource and policy initiative.

Policy initiative, as well as the recognition of fathers *per se*, nonetheless touches upon some fundamental issues about the value attributed to active parenting by fathers, both among policy makers and among health professionals.

If it is attitudes to and recognition of fathers, rather than expertise in new information content, that makes most of the difference to the messages that they take away from the processes of health professionals and service environments before and after the birth of their children, it is worth examining such attitudes, values and recognition in some detail.

For this reason, questions relevant to these issues are explored in Chapters 2 and 3 before turning, in Chapter 4, to more specific aspects of methods of information design and delivery that are both inclusive of and accessible to fathers. However, it is also argued that answering fathers' information needs implicitly acts as recognition of their parenting, which is beneficial in itself. It is argued that these benefits extend to mothers and children as well as to the men involved.

The particular receptiveness of men around the time of the birth argues for the benefits of recognising and supporting fathers' parenting both before and after the birth itself. This involves more than the methods of engaging fathers that are sometimes currently used in the delivery room, which can be applied from the moment the father first attends an antenatal appointment to the last postnatal visit by the health visitor. Beyond this, projects that seek to support fathers' parenting may benefit by considering some of the issues raised in Chapter 4 about reaching men and designing services for them.

The evidence of fathers' receptiveness around the time of the birth already seems to be broadly accepted. The NFPI survey itself posits the value of 'targeting men proactively when they are receptive (e.g. at the birth)', and Trefor Lloyd, following Emma Longstaff, cites James Levine's highlighting of the birth as providing a golden opportunity to access men:

> She reinforces the need to identify primary motivation, saying that: Levine and others have observed certain moments in fathers' lives offer golden moments for intervention, such as the birth of a child or, more unhappily, divorce. Agencies who have contact with families at these times should be certain to make the most of these golden opportunities, and design their services accordingly.[5]

It appears that the effect which this receptiveness has is to increase the likelihood of the father bonding with his newborn child – provided that this golden opportunity is capitalised on. For example, Dr Anthony Clare highlights the effect of men being given the opportunity to hold their newborn children:

> In a study of 45 infants delivered by Caesarean section, half were presented to the father to hold for 10 minutes, while the other half were put in incubators, the fathers only being allowed to visit and look, not touch. At three months, those fathers who had held their babies were much more involved with their infants than those who had not.[6]

One means of taking advantage of the opportunities to involve fathers at this time is by designing accessible baby-care courses that include information for men who are about to become fathers. These, too, have been found to have measurable effects in promoting involvement, as Lewis has described:

> Fathers who had participated in baby-care courses undertook more care of their babies than fathers who had not, and they also kept closer to

them and engaged in more face-to-face interaction with them. At nine months, the babies of these fathers were said to be 'happier'.[7]

In bonding men with their families, the opportunity may also arise to offer positive approaches and messages to men with regard to a socially positive engagement instead of the corrective and negative messages about fathers' relationships with women and children that have thus far been the focus of attention. It will be argued later in this book that such negative messages tend to undermine fathers' positive engagement with their families and children, if they are not counterbalanced with positive messages.

Clare illustrates the social benefits of engaged fatherhood as follows:

> Analysing patterns over four decades of male life, Snarey found that men who took an active role in the home were, by the time their children were grown, better managers, community leaders and role models. He found, too, that the amount and quality of their care for their children's social and emotional development during childhood and adolescence actually predicted the fathers' later marital stability and contentment. The more fathers participated in the rearing of their children during early adulthood, the more likely these fathers were to be happily married at midlife.[8]

However, the implications of offering men other identities do not just bear upon men, and should not be regarded as merely another opportunity to admonish men for failing in their relationships with women and society. There is equally the opportunity for women to look at ways of facilitating fathers' engagement in families, particularly when so many rely on this engagement to allow them to be active in the workplace. As Williams has expressed it, again emphasising the opportunity presented by the birth:

> becoming a parent provides a golden opportunity for men, and women, to examine their roles and identities. Those opportunities are equally there for practitioners and services to work effectively with fathers if strategy, resources and reflexive methods are developed.[9]

The implications for women were also addressed by Professor Howard Dubowitz in an interview with *The Sunday Times* in which his research findings of the benefits to children of involved fathers were discussed:

> What we have is the strong suggestion that kids benefit from having a man around, and they especially benefit if the man is loving and supportive. The $64 000 question is how we can engage these men and have them involved in their kids' lives.
> [He warned:] It also says something to the women: I see well-meaning, well-educated professional women who in subtle or not so subtle ways discourage men from being involved. In various ways mothers have unwittingly discouraged men. When, for example, both parents bring in kids to see the doctor there is an assumption that the woman has all the information, and not the father.

These might seem like small things, but in an era when we are trying to get men to play bigger and better roles in family life, that kind of thing doesn't help.[10]

In the re-examination of roles and identities, it is worth noting that there may be something of a premium in identifying first-time fathers, as attendance at antenatal classes drops off among second-time or more fathers, indicating that patterns of parenting among couples may tend to be set by a first child.

References

1 Office of National Statistics (1999) *Labour Force Survey*. Office of National Statistics, London.
2 Gingerbread (2001) *Becoming Visible: focus on lone fathers.* Action Facts. Gingerbread, London, p. 1.
3 National Family and Parenting Institute (2001) *National Mapping of Family Support Services in England and Wales*. National Family and Parenting Institute, London.
4 Buchanan A and Flouri E (2001) *Father Involvement and Outcomes in Adolescence and Adulthood*. ESRC End of Award Report R000223309. Department of Social Policy and Social Work, Oxford University, p. 1.
5 Lloyd T (2001) *What Works with Fathers?* Working With Men, London, citing Longstaff E (2000) *Fathers Figure: fathers' groups in family policy*. Institute for Public Policy Research, London.
6 Clare A (2000) *On Men: masculinity in crisis*. Chatto & Windus, London, p. 180, citing Roedholm M (1981) Effect of father–infant postpartum contact in their interaction 3 months after birth. *Early Hum Dev.* **5**: 79–85.
7 *FatherFacts. Volume 1, Issue 1* (2001) Fathers Direct, Newpin Fathers Support Centre, NFPI and Working With Men, footnote 8, p. 9, citing Nickel H and Kocher EMT (1987) West Germany and the German speaking countries. In: ME Lamb (ed.) *The Father's Role. Cross Cultural Perspectives*. Lawrence Erlbaum, New Jersey.
8 Clare, op. cit., p. 172.
9 Williams R (1999) *Going the Distance: fathers, health and health visiting*. University of Reading in association with the Queen's Nursing Institute, London, p. 25.
10 Dobson R (2000) Children with father in family have a head start in life. *Sunday Times*. **21 May**.

CHAPTER 2

A male role model: for children, mothers – and men?

Why focus on the value of fathers?

> - Attitudes of workers to men and fathers can determine whether fathers are given recognition as potentially involved parents.
> - Where workers' attitudes to men tend to be negative, those attitudes are often based on socially negative behaviour by men.

From assessments of what approaches are successful when working with men, top of the list appears to be project workers and staff members having a fundamentally positive attitude to men and valuing what they can bring to children and their families.

If health professionals value men in this way, they will be able to adapt their skills to meet the needs of the individual father in much the same way as they adapt them to meet the needs of the individual mother. The need is for the basic valuing of men to underlie all communication with them. For this reason it is worth looking at the value of fathers at some length, as well as considering how father-hood might be valuable to men.

In March 2001, the National Council of Voluntary Child Care Organisations (NCVCCO), as part of its Supporting Families Project, held a conference entitled *Are We Shutting Out Fathers?*

The conference made eight recommendations, of which the first four were as follows.

1 Female workers should look at and examine their attitudes to fathers and men.
2 Training courses/sessions should be established for all members of staff and volunteers about self-awareness and working with fathers/men. They should include workers in family centres, nurseries, family support agencies in both voluntary and statutory sectors, health visitors, social workers, midwives, etc. (all of whom are predominantly female).
3 Family support agencies should make an effort to become more welcoming to men/fathers and to be more aware of the environment. For example, they

should have posters and photos portraying positive images of men as fathers, and magazines relating to 'male' hobbies (e.g. fishing, sports, cars, etc.) as well as the usual parenting magazines.

4   Agencies and organisations should become more inclusive of fathers and be aware of the difficulties that men have in entering an all-female environment.[1]

This conference identified the attitudes of workers to men and fathers as a common barrier towards working positively with men and fathers and supporting families effectively. There are a number of reasons for arguing why moving forward from such entrenched positions would actually help to solve the perceived problems with regard to aspects of men's behaviour.

Enabling a positive masculinity: socialising male role models

- This section, which is divided into subsections below, deals with the need for men to be offered a wider range of socially positive identities (e.g. involved fatherhood which engages them in society and benefits women and children), tending to focus less on their status as breadwinners at a time when changing patterns of employment, women's access to the workplace and changing families make the unique breadwinning role of the father too narrow a foundation upon which to base a socially engaged masculinity available to men.

The value to men of being involved fathers: a random note

- Later in life, fathers can strongly regret their lack of involvement with their children if they did not get involved from the outset.

Listeners to BBC Radio 4 will know that from time to time it broadcasts distress calls – urgent messages from family members who have lost touch with each other for some time, even in this era of email and the mobile phone. Some may have noticed a pattern – very often these messages are addressed to sons 'last known to be living' in one area or another about their father 'who is dangerously ill'. Fathers who have lost touch with their children seem to make disproportionate use of this desperate means of making contact with them as their final act before they die. It seems sad that for these fathers at the end of their lives, as for so many others, they should so often regret the missed opportunities to be involved with their children.

On the other hand, a measure of the intrinsic need for children to at least count on having a father figure would seem to be found in the search by adoptees for their biological parents. Daniel and Taylor refer to the father providing a sense of 'socio-genealogical connectedness' informing them of their culture and heritage. A similar measure would also seem to be found in the pain and anguish that are experienced by those who have lost their fathers.

But what might be the benefits of a more active parenting identity for the fathers themselves?

The confusion surrounding masculinity for fathers

- The relationship between male care for children and masculinity is undefined for both male childcare workers and fathers.
- The breadwinner role still has force, but within the family, although the remote disciplinarian model is no longer regarded as satisfactory, the fully involved father model is seldom encouraged as an alternative.
- Fathers appear to have a strength as playmates, but this can be viewed as too permissive an approach to children, whereas the disciplinarian approach can be seen as excessively prescriptive.
- Fathers taking the 'playmate' role are subject to the criticism that they are 'creaming off' the most enjoyable aspects of childcare, whereas this role is well defined for them.

With regard to media representations, there is confusion about the perceived mainstream identities for parents. For women, the mainstream identity is the stay-at-home married mother. The media does not seem to have caught up with changing attitudes about having children outside marriage reflected recently by the Eighteenth British Social Attitudes Survey.[2] Either opprobrium is heaped upon working mothers, who are deemed to be neglectful of their children, or else single mothers, constrained by the lack of affordable childcare to living on State benefits, are deemed to be neglectful of their responsibilities to the economy.

Despite the contradictory fact that in practice many stay-at-home mothers feel significant societal pressure to become income earners, their position as the standard bearer or kitemark of mainstream female parent identity remains substantially secure.

Yet there is no such kitemark identity for fathers. If they adhere to the distant breadwinning patriarchal model, they are perceived as being remote as parents and out of touch with modern values. Yet as an alternative, there is much confusion surrounding the nurturing involved father and little definition of his role. Often it seems to be confined to a partial aspect of involvement – the role of playmate. Although this role is one of the best defined for fathers, and is further outlined in the subsection below dealing with the value to children of involved fathers (*see* p. 39), it is often reduced to the concept that fathers should play football with their sons. The emphasis on sons and football can moreover be seen to speak of an implicit confusion (as well as some apprehensions) about their involvement with their daughters.

Thus whatever variety exists in real life, there is a perceived mainstream role identity for mothers, but not for fathers. Judged by the value attributed to their breadwinning and thus the long-hours culture at work, they nonetheless have been reported to feel under pressure to be 'superdads',[3] enjoying great relationships with their children, but without the time to develop them. For non-income-earning fathers, the predominance of the breadwinning role daily undermines the value which they feel that they can bring to their children by being involved and present parents.

The value of a new masculine identity of involved fatherhood

- Men need to be offered a wider range of positive identities to reflect and draw on the strengths of their real diversity.
- Involved fatherhood is one such socially positive identity for men, and it can help to expand the meaning of masculinity in a positive direction.
- Workers can help to connect men with this socially positive identity at the time of the birth.
- Fathers' actual involvement can be underestimated, often by men themselves. Workers can help to connect existing positive behaviour by men with masculinity by recognising and acknowledging positive behaviour.
- Such recognition could help to establish a shared vocabulary of parenting for men.

A random note is added here. In Disney's animated films, just as the predominance of men made muscular by their work is diminishing as the need for unskilled manual labour declines, the ideal body type of the hero is becoming more muscular. Compare the prince in *Snow White* (1937) with the one in *Beauty and the Beast* (1991).

Men are publicly obliged to adopt, through lack of choice and alternatives, a narrow definition of masculinity (muscular, economically powerful/breadwinner) that flies in the face of their real diversity and does not reflect the relative lack of opportunities today for them fully to exercise that narrow definition. The laws of supply and demand seem to be driving up the value of an ever scarcer commodity – a version of masculinity that is in reality dwindling. In adding to their body bulk, men are compensating for their relative impotence in reality as economic power is transferred to women.

Yet this is not always simply a story of unemployment among men. What it can be is a pattern of sharing income earning between men and women. This is particularly important when pay rates are lower in the modern service economy than in the old male-dominated manufacturing sector. It is not always recognised that sharing income earning can also mean sharing the childcare. Research for Children North East revealed that unemployment:

> though still higher than average in the region, was not the predominant pattern. More obvious was that mothers and fathers were juggling

low-paid shift work in order to share the care of their children. And yet in spite of this there is, still, substantial prejudice in professional circles about men as carers.[4]

These developments peak into real crisis when they impose a terrible burden on boys and young men whose values are forged by narrowing expectations of masculinity that do not reflect changes such as those in employment patterns, but who are offered only condemnation and ostracisation (sometimes from professionals) should they seek to question or depart from them. They are offered neither alternative role models nor support in identifying and voicing their concerns. The result is an epidemic of suicide among boys and young men.[5]

I say that men – and here I am talking about fathers – are nominally subscribing to a single definition of masculinity. By this it is meant that they do so in public. Take a closer look, however, and what is found is that fathers are not an homogenous group.[6] They differ individually in a multitude of ways from the perceived kitemark of masculine identity.

In practice, this presents the difficulty (which we shall examine shortly) that there is no one way of accessing them. How do you access the private individual father? But as well as measures of health professionals' practice, there are broader gains to be obtained by promoting a socially constructive masculinity.

Although fathers vary as individuals, they are nonetheless conscious of where they might be perceived to vary from the kitemark, and apparently sensitive about it. Although many fathers collect their children from school, it does not seem that when they are doing so they acknowledge each other in the way that mothers do. Fathers with children in public places often do not make eye contact with each other. It seems as if they both think of fatherhood as an activity that is not within the stereotypically permitted shared templates of masculine interactions such as sport, cars, sex or drink. Outside the boundaries of these shared templates it seems that men – even these men who are engaged in a similar activity – have no shared vocabulary with which to address each other. The effect of fathers thus playing down their involvement in public tends to make them invisible to service providers as caring parents,[7] but it is also a feature of men being boxed into an extremely narrow range of permitted identities.

Surely there must be a value in promoting positive parenting by fathers as a version of masculinity that men can aspire to – and acknowledge among themselves. If there is such a value, there must be benefits in this context if health professionals acknowledge the fathers whom they encounter. Equally, recognition by health professionals will tend to promote such self-acknowledgement among fathers.

It is essential that this range of identities be expanded for men's socially positive interaction with society, in contrast to the ever-broadening range of socially destructive identities that the unassimilated male can assume, and in contrast to the ever-narrowing permitted range of the kitemark male identity.

In the subsection on barriers to father involvement (*see* p. 51) factors that inhibit fathers' involvement with their children and the ways men perceive fatherhood as an ideal are examined in detail. However, a major inhibition or barrier to men's involvement with their children is currently to be found in the prevalence of the stereotype of the father as abuser.

The focus on aberrant masculinities: child abuse

> • Generalised societal concerns about child abuse should not prevent workers from encouraging involved fatherhood.
> • Campaigns against child abuse may be having a broadly adverse effect on men's involvement with children.
> • Fathers who do not have positive relationships with their children may be more likely to pose a threat.

Dr Anthony Clare in *Masculinity in Crisis* makes the point that:

> concern is now being raised that just as more men have been persuaded of the benefits for them, their partners and their children of greater participation by fathers in the care and development of their children, the spectre of child sexual abuse has made men fearful of getting too close to their children, especially daughters, and anxious about the expression of affection.[8]

The concern that fears about child abuse are boxing men into a narrow public masculinity that does not admit childcare responsibilities is probably well founded, but difficult to prove in the case of individual fathers. What father would say that campaigns against child abuse, which often focus on abusive men and fathers, have compromised his enjoyment of family life? He would be aware of the perception that he was admitting to abusive behaviour – just as if he said it had not. However, there is some evidence of the way in which fathers' involvement with their families has been damaged. For example, Burgess quotes a father of two:[9]

> [Phil, a father of two (two families)] In autumn 1990, I was walking up the Holloway Road with my mate, and we were both carrying our babies in slings on our chests. This car went past with these young blokes in it, and they slowed right down, rolled down the windows, and yelled out 'Child abusers!'. Nothing like that happened 16 years ago when I was going round with my first son, doing much the same things. I think attitudes have changed. I think some men are scared to be seen being intimate with their children.

Also, as Rick Marin reported about a home-dad convention in the *New York Times*:

> Experiences of a so-called 'glass wall' separating mothers from fathers in parks and schoolyards echoed around the room. Edward Howard, 54, said, 'I go to the playground with my son and I'm tired of being looked at as some kind of sexual pervert.'[10]

Furthermore, a report by the Daycare Trust found that men are reluctant to enter the childcare workforce because they 'are worried about being accused of child abuse',[11] and a report on lone fathers for the charity Gingerbread found that 'The publicity given to child abuse … has also affected many men with caring and responsible attitudes to working with or bringing up children.'[12]

The Gingerbread report acknowledges the effect of the publicity given to child abuse on both fathers and men working with children. As soon as a father leaves the home with his children, his parenting becomes a public form of childcare by men, just like that of a primary schoolteacher. Therefore if men are found to be withdrawing from public forms of childcare, such as teaching, the same mechanisms must operate with the effect that fathers withdraw from involvement with and displays of affection towards their children, fearing perceptions and misplaced accusations of abuse, particularly in public. This withdrawal from the public sphere will tend to compound the invisibility of their parenting.

In primary schools the numbers of male teachers is now at crisis level. They are absent in a large number of primary schools, and the Government has admitted that there is a worrying shortage of male role models in the classroom.[13] There are a variety of causes for this development, including historic levels of pay. However, as the *Independent* reported recently, 'many argue that the money is no longer the real issue.' In the same report, Professor John Howson, an expert on teacher recruitment:

> puts much of the blame for the decline of male applicants on the child protection legislation that came in after the 1989 Children Act. 'We had a lot of societal unease about men in the caring profession (*sic*) that we have probably worked through now. We have good checks in place, and there is no reason men shouldn't work as well with young children as women.'[14]

The Gingerbread report's *action facts* supplement drew attention specifically to the effect of negative stereotyping on fathers in making the recommendation that 'All those involved in the policy debate and media should be aware of the impact of negative stereotyping of both lone parents *and fathers*[15] as a contributory factor to social exclusion for both lone fathers and their children.'

It must be emphasised that it is imperative, as a matter of principle, to promote child safety and prevent abuse. Men must acknowledge abusive behaviour where they are found to perpetrate it – and, tragically, it occurs all too often.

However, it must be considered that child protection messages – finding fertile ground in stereotypes of abusive male behaviour, giving an unbalanced picture of men's involvement with their families, and concentrating on a corrective–coercive approach – may tend to undermine men's positive interaction with their children and families as much as they inhibit abusive behaviour in families where such abuse occurs or is at risk of occurring. Messages that portray fathers uniquely as perpetrators will tend to undermine the value that the father perceives is attributed to his proper parenting. Undermining the father's perception of the value of his parenting cannot be of benefit to his family.

An example of the need for such positive messages to balance corrective ones is perhaps to be found in the Government campaign launched in April 2002 in an attempt to persuade more men to become primary teachers. By this time only 14.4% of primary teachers were men.[16] The damage done to father involvement is less easy to quantify.

If he is unsure of his value to his family, a father may become alienated from his family. In such circumstances there is a hypothetical risk that the father's behaviour towards the family will tend to become alien itself. It is a further possibility that messages that do not reinforce the potential value of the father as a positive figure, as well as taking a corrective approach to negative behaviour, may be implicated in indirectly preparing the ground for abusive behaviour.

Men in the nursery: which role model for workers and fathers?

- The debate about the value of men as childcare workers acts as a key to values that are held about fathers.
- Uncertainty about whether such men are there to challenge or reinforce gender stereotypes reflects uncertainty about the direction that fatherhood should take.
- Generalised fears of sexual abuse pervade the debate, but it is not clear whether such fears about men and child abuse lead to the regressive notion that childcare is women's work, or whether they stem from that notion.
- Different expectations apply to men's caring.
- 'Fears about abuse' thus tend to move men's caring away from nurturing and towards less physically close types of engagement such as play.
- Workers should not impose prescriptive models/their own expectations of fatherhood on families, just as with motherhood, but rather they should work with the strengths of individual fathers and partnerships.

It has been noted above that the 'ideal' father figure is less well defined than the 'ideal' mother figure (however restrictive that may be for women), tending as it does to swing between the poles of rigid disciplinarian and over-permissive playmate, neither of which is itself found to be satisfactory.

Much emphasis is put on the role of the father as provider or breadwinner – often by men themselves – but there seems to be less overall certainty about how he should interact with his family, and with his children in particular, when he is present. This is despite the fact that the value to children of involved father-hood has been profoundly researched by some academics, notably Lamb (and is addressed later in this book). Issues of this kind have, on the other hand, been made somewhat more explicit in the context of the debate about men working with children – that is, male childcare workers. This is perhaps because although fatherhood as studied by Lamb and others is a given (albeit often remaining unascertained), the choice of recruiting a male childcare worker presents itself as an option that is open for public debate.

The debate has focused on the value or otherwise that male childcare workers can bring to children. Often the debate is focused on the perceived threat that men pose to children, particularly in relation to sexual abuse. However, it has had the effect of throwing a sidelight on to the perceived value that fathers can bring to children as men caring for children. *Men in the Nursery* is the title of a book by Cameron, Moss and Owen which explored and researched these issues.[17]

In essence what was found by Cameron and her colleagues was broad agree-ment that there should be more male childcare workers than the current negligible number, but there is a more profound disagreement over the reasons why this level should be increased. Thus although the Department for Education and Employment has a target of 6% for men in the childcare workforce, this will almost certainly remain a mere aspiration until there is a greater concensus. Essentially the different reasons for increasing the male childcare workforce polarise around the mutually exclusive rationales of whether the men should be there to challenge or to reinforce gender stereotypes. It is often said that men should be present in the nursery as a 'role model'. However, what often remains unclear is what type of role model is intended. Some regard the presence of men in the nursery as an opportunity to incubate 'new man', while others focus on the importance of emphasising the dis-tinct roles of men and women to children from the earliest age. So on the surface, for example, a wish to have more men involved in 'childcare', although sounding progressive, can mean that it is intended that the men remain within explicitly masculine modalities of childcare, particularly outdoor play. Others (notably child-care course lecturers) express a wish to see more men in childcare in order to pro-vide children with more progressive models of men and women working together.

However, although nearly all parents expressly wished to see more male childcare workers, mainly in order to demonstrate that caring is not just women's work, in practice parents reacted with resistance, suspicion, hostility, or in some cases exaggerated welcome to seeing men in the nursery. About a third of the parents who were interviewed by Cameron and her colleagues identified some potential disadvantages of employing male workers. Virtually all of these involved assumptions made by wider society about sexual abuse. What arises here is another example of public aspirations for men and children conflicting with relatively pri-vate apprehensions about them – the subject of child abuse being an uncom-fortable issue to discuss publicly. Nonetheless, as Daniel and Taylor have observed about structural forces in society which can act as barriers to fatherhood, 'the failure to examine these forces and how they impact on the individual explains why simple exhortations to men to be more involved have minimal effect and, of course, why simple exhortations to practitioners to engage with fathers have minimal effect.'[18] Thus although Claire Cameron has argued for dispelling on a national scale the idea that male workers and abuse are necessarily linked,[19] until such a decoupling is promoted nationally in this way, aspirations for 6% of the childcare workforce to consist of men will remain as such, particularly in the absence of a fundamental consensus as to whether they are there to challenge or reinforce gender stereo-types. The idea that all men are abusive is of course a gender stereotype in itself, so among those who would argue for the validity of such stereotypes prevailing in all individual instances there will be no wish to hire a male childcare worker from the outset.

Thus although there is a generalised express wish to increase the male childcare workforce in order to demonstrate that caring is not just women's work, some aspects of fears about child abuse may appear to be having the regressive effect of reinforcing the expectation that childcare is, properly, just that – women's work. What is not always so clear is whether this reinforcement arises from cause or effect. That is to say it is less clear, when in general many gender divides are dis-appearing, whether generalised fears about men and child abuse lead to the regres-sive notion that childcare is women's work, or whether they stem from that notion.

Closer analysis of what forms male caring should 'ideally' take reveals differences in expectations between men's and women's caring, and forms of childcare which tend to reveal a resistance to and ignorance of nurturing by men. As Cameron and her colleagues' research revealed:

> Different expectations for men and women also emerged when we examined the allocation of work in the centres. While women reported that there were no differences between men and women in allocation of work, men found they were often expected to undertake practical or heavy work such as maintenance, and were expected to like particular forms of play, such as football and playing with trucks and cars. We concluded that the experience of being a man, particularly where he worked as a minority of one or two, could be described as marginalised.[20]

The source of these expectations may be in part due to the way in which Nursery Nursing and Early Childhood studies are taught. Cameron and colleagues found that:

> the female gender is absolutely integral to the way the courses are taught and the way students and staff are thought about. The staff find it difficult to present an alternative viewpoint to their own (female) gender; the female students 'mother' the male students; and the discourse that is employed emphasises the femaleness of the caring role.[21]

It appears, then, that there is a greater emphasis in practice on men being in the nursery in order to reinforce gender stereotypes rather than to challenge them.

The fact that male workers often work in a minority of one or two promotes a message or stereotype of its own (notably challenged by Sheffield Children's Centre, where men and women are present in equal proportion) that men are of relatively marginal significance, particularly to young children.

Where the femaleness of the caring role is the prevailing latent assumption in childcare courses, it is possible to see fears about child abuse as a kind of catalyst which, when added to that assumption, promote a specific reaction against caring (or nurturing) by men. In this sense it is possible to argue that generalised fears about men and child abuse stem from the regressive notion that childcare is women's work more than they lead to it. Fears about abuse thus tend to move men's caring away from nurturing and towards less physically close types of engagement in play (often outdoors, where it can be observed). The emphasis on men's strengths in play itself then tends to promote the underlying assumption about the risks posed by their caring or nurturing in a reinforcing cycle.

As has been noted earlier, the lack of clarity in the debate about what 'type' of male childcare worker is the ideal (although, in practice, expectations tend to coalesce around 'masculine' play behaviours or activities) is reflected in a similar lack of clarity with regard to expectations of the 'ideal' father. However, it was suggested in the previous section that apprehension about perceptions of abuse may be having a similarly adverse effect on fathers' caring to that on male childcare workers in so far as fathers may be apprehensive about showing any displays of affection towards their children. It may be that fathers are also moving towards 'approved' forms of play, rather than expressing affection overtly. However, there is one clear difference between fathers and male childcare workers. It has been noted that the absence of agreement about the strengths of male childcare workers contributes to their low levels of recruitment, but for fathers recruitment is not the issue. On the other hand, how to support fathers' parenting may be seen as a valid question. Here the issue is about what exactly practitioners should be supporting – much as the question about male childcare workers is about which type of care is regarded as appropriate to the circumstances.

Daniel and Taylor suggest that 'Practitioners need to be clear about what roles they envisage fathers playing in their children's lives',[22] and they go on to suggest that these may include four specific roles which they can perform – of partnership (traditional or non-traditional, i.e. breadwinner/carer or shared parenting) with the mother, alternative mother (father as primary or principal carer), luxury (which they define as a kind of 'add-on' assistant) or a unique role (outside the integrated family). Nonetheless, they are careful also to suggest that practitioners anticipate the role which the father himself considers to be appropriate. Although these may be seen as valuable practice points in being more inclusive towards fathers, it is perhaps important to develop the point that 'ideal' roles, once defined, should not be imposed upon fathers in the way that the stay-at-home nurturing model was once (and still is) imposed in many respects on mothers. Rather, they should perhaps act as sketch 'route maps' to assist the father in playing the role that he himself (as Daniel and Taylor say) considers to be appropriate.

What is implied as a vital ingredient in this process is for the professional to enter into a dialogue with the father. Reflecting the point made above that route maps should be distinct from orthodox imposed models of fathering, Daniel and Taylor do also make it clear that 'Supporting families should take place within the family's own notions of fatherhood, traditional or non-traditional, not the practitioner's.' Again there is an important point to develop here, which is perhaps found in the emphasis on the concept of the family. That is to say, it may equally be beneficial to find out from the mother what she considers to be appropriate with her own parenting, and thereby to discover and build upon her strengths, perhaps using model 'route maps' as a guide, just as described above for the father. Equally important are the couple's expectations of each other. Other family members such as grandparents may also come into the picture. Working with the father in complete isolation, as health professionals currently tend to do with the mother, and using models of care appropriate to one kind of motherhood or fatherhood alone (e.g. full-time, primary carer mother) must be regarded as equally unsatisfactory.

It is perhaps important to suggest here that in 'discovering' the field of fatherhood, practitioners may consider that the context of the parents' relationship is just as important as considerations of gender pertaining to the individual parents. In some cases (traditional breadwinner/carer) they may each have neatly fitting gendered ideas of each other's roles formed by sex role expectations, but in other cases these expectations may not be shared, or the couple may have fashioned their own expectations of each other and reached a mutually satisfactory understanding. It is such an understanding between the parents that is perhaps the ideal for the practitioner to attempt to steer towards, by comparing 'route maps' or otherwise facilitating a dialogue between the parents about how they are jointly to approach their parenting. This suggestion is explored further below in the sections dealing with the father's oft repeated 'supporter role' at the time of the birth.

It is also worth bearing in mind that as far as their children's needs are con-cerned, there are as many *potentially* valid ways of being a father as there are fathers. Obviously in a few cases that potential will be marred by violence or abuse. However, men as well as fathers are more varied than is often recognised. What this means is that good (or potentially good) fathering can take many forms according to the individual father and the circumstances in which he finds himself, rather than in prescribed models. The father may simply need an endorsement of the direction in which he is already moving and an acknowledgement of his parenthood to boost his self-confidence and subsequent acquisition of skills.

Practitioners may reasonably be wary of facilitating dialogue between parents if there is any sign of conflict, for fear of being drawn into a mediating role for which they are not equipped. It is as important to have the skills to close down a discus-sion positively as it is to be able to open it up, and these skills are only acquired by training. It is ultimately for the parents to negotiate and evolve their own part-nership in parenting between themselves. Depending on the circumstances, it may be simply desirable for practitioners who are beginning to work with fathers as well as mothers to ensure that they are careful to include the father in discussions and accord him the same recognition as a parent and as a resource for the child as they do the mother.

It is in this context that the concept of involved fatherhood referred to in this book is not specifically defined in a prescriptive way, but broadly refers to an interaction and presence with the child, and perhaps the family, that is widely beneficial and should therefore be encouraged.

Does supporting fathers mean undermining mothers?

- Supporting fathers' involvement with families should be a part of working with the family holistically as a mutually supporting unit, rather than prioritising parenting by fathers or mothers.
- Such an approach, which emphasises the value of relationships, reduces the likelihood of relationship breakdown.
- Healthy relationships between parents benefit children's development.
- Supporting fathers' involvement should not be perceived to undermine single motherhood. The vast majority of single mothers want involved fathers.

It is an occupational hazard for people who support fathers' involvement in the family that their work is sometimes seen as necessarily undermining mothers and thus inherently misogynistic. However, this view could not be more wrong. Facilitating what fathers can bring to their families *supports mothers* both in and out of the home – both as parents and at work. And the 'involvement' of their partner with the family and children is put at a premium by many mothers.[23]

Much public acrimony about relationships between the sexes arises from the bit-terness of relationship breakdown. This bitterness becomes magnified by the polar-isation that is caused by the adversarial divorce process. The legal process is a major source of perceptions that a gain for one 'side' must mean a loss for the other. Thus the 'gender war' becomes a zero sum game.

However, supporting fathers' parenting and involving the father in the family makes divorce and separation *much less likely*, as Adrienne Burgess noted in *Fatherhood Reclaimed*:[24]

> In the US, Caroline and Philip Cowan have evaluated group counselling for expectant couples .... After 18 months, the prepared parents were showing more flexibility in work and family arrangements than the unprepareds, and the prepared fathers were more satisfied about everything than the unprepared fathers, including their partner's parenting. But the most significant of all was the fact that while one out of every eight of the *un*prepared couples had split up (together with one out of six of a comparison sample of childless couples), there was not one relationship breakdown among the prepared couples. They were *all* still together, as they were two years on, when the Cowans interviewed them again, and when another unprepared couple had parted.

And outcomes for children are better if there are two parents present. However, this touches on an area of contention as to why this might be.

Particular difficulty stems from assumptions that supporting fathers' involvement in families and with their children is calculated to undermine single mothers. Contention focuses on the question of whether poorer outcomes for children of single-parent households are attributable to the absence of the father or to the lower household incomes of single-parent families. The quality of single mothers' parenting is deemed to be at issue, and blame is deemed to be attributable to their parenting if poorer outcomes for their children are said to exist. Thus their parenting is viewed from the same deficit perspective as fathers' parenting.

However, widowed, separated and divorced mothers – the majority by far – did not choose to have children on their own. Like most mothers, they wanted involved fathers.

Setting fathers and single mothers against each other is like asking them to compete for last prize in a race that no one should be encouraging. Both have their own value to their children. However, if there is a father around in a specific case, it makes sense to support his parenting and unlock his potential as a carer. There is also the argument that 'a father who stays is a father who pays'. This answers the household income point, and is attractive to governments that are seeking to reduce welfare costs, but it casts the father firmly in the breadwinner role and tends to diminish his potential as a carer.

The distinction must also be made between supporting fathers and supporting marriage. The recent Eighteenth British Social Attitudes Survey[25] showed clear acceptance (46% overall, rising to two-thirds (66%) among the 18- to 24-year-old age group) for parenthood outside marriage. In our society, parenthood and marriage no longer necessarily go together.

Much of the historic controversy about divorce has focused on the damage that is said to be done to the children. This has been a hotly debated area. However, the debate has concentrated on the question of long-term effects. What is not at issue is the fact that the process of relationship breakdown is usually a miserable experience for the children at the time. It is also recognised as being an adverse environment for children's development, whether headlined by a formal divorce or not. As Burgess puts it, 'the single most important indicator of maladjustment in children is their parents' active hostility – to each other.'[26] If a relatively small input into facilitating the father's parenting can have the effects that are observed in reducing relationship breakdown, as the Cowans found, it must be of benefit in reducing the misery that is experienced by children due to the breakdown of their parents' relationship and the adverse outcomes that can stem from this.

Do mothers want involved fathers, or do they just want support?

- Practitioners sometimes take the view that it is for the mother to determine the father's level of involvement, and they may exclude the father for this reason.
- However, promoting the father's involvement within the context of the parents' relationship and both their expectations builds on the strength of both parents and relieves the burden on mothers.
- It is perhaps equally important that mothers should not be burdened with the suggestion that a good mother essentially copes alone. This suggestion is implicit in the father being ignored as a potentially equal partner in parenting.
- If the father's role in some cases is deemed to be that of a supporter, he must at least be given the information and support to enable him to fulfil this task.
- Mothers appear to want a varying mixture of support and involvement, but support in the long term becomes a feature of involvement.

Every so often the findings of a survey are published in which the vast majority of mothers surveyed express the wish for more support with childcare and household duties in the home from their partners.[27] Editorials criticise fathers for underperforming and not getting involved, with headlines about 'slack dads' – an idea that is now so ingrained that one columnist uses this as the title of his occasional articles, with no apparent trace of irony. The Joseph Rowntree Foundation study entitled *Fathers, Work and Family Life*[28] found that although most fathers identified their role with regard to the children as provider, in contrast most mothers indeed wanted fathers to be involved. However, this study and others[29] have shown that 'involvement' can have a variety of meanings, ranging from the father undertaking activities and forging relationships with the children, to lesser degrees of involvement such as 'being there' or simply 'being available'.

Thus the type of involvement that is desired can be seen to exist on a continuum, with more direct involvement being wanted at one end of the scale, and 'being available' towards the other end. At the outer end of this continuum, studies identifying five principal barriers to father involvement have identified the fact that 'Women who become full-time mothers might think their role is threatened and the balance of matrimonial power has shifted if their partners become too active or skilled in childcare.'[30] The father's role as breadwinner and provider, in contrast to his involvement within the dynamics of the family, is much clearer and as the studies have shown men are particularly conscious of the perceived value of the role.

Thus it appears that some mothers may even tend actively to resist father involvement and can experience difficulty in managing potentially competing desires – for support from their partners on the one hand, and a need to be the axial point of the family on the other. As the studies have found, 'women have strong feelings against abdicating their role as primary caretakers of their babies.' As is further outlined in Chapter 4 on reaching fathers, mothers have been found to act as 'gatekeepers', moderating the level of father involvement in the family. As has already been noted, this appears to apply particularly to full-time mothers.

By way of illustration, a similar situation may be said to apply when women earn as much or more than their partners, thereby encroaching on the man's traditional role as provider and breadwinner. For some men this appears to be a difficulty, while for others it poses no problem. It appears that men have varying attitudes to their supposed principal function being encroached upon, or shared – just as women apparently do. However, most of the time it is necessity that determines the need for shared income earning and therefore shared childcare.

Ongoing research by Penelope Leach for the National Child Minders Association (NCMA), in which mothers were asked, when their children were three months old, what they thought would be the ideal form of childcare if money was no object, has found that grandparents were top of the list for mothers who considered that care provided by someone other than themselves would be ideal. Fathers were the least favoured option, with less than 1% of mothers wanting the father to be the carer.[31] About half of the mothers wanted to care for their babies themselves and did so. In practice, in Leach's findings, nearly one in ten fathers was looking after the children at 12 months of age.

Leach's research starts by asking mothers to hypothesise about an ideal, but it reveals a strong attachment by mothers to a principal role in care for young children, and to models of care by others that replicate their own. However, it also reveals that mothers' adaptation to real conditions can modify their outlook. Entrenched assumptions that are held at the outset may therefore be of limited value.

Thus when the readers of a mothering magazine or website (often the source of the surveys mentioned above) are asked whether they want fathers to become more involved with childcare, the positive response is anywhere between 60% and 80%. However, add to this aspiration the conjectured real-world cost of ceding their unique bond with the child and their place at the axial point of the family (as is implied by Leach's suggestion that the father be the full-time or principal carer), and the positive response is less than 1%. Variations of this degree render these surveys or survey components almost meaningless. They can only signify that real-world factors – such as the need for two incomes – have a very significant bearing on what people want in reality. Leach's research shows that experience has significantly modified the outlook of many of its respondents. What practitioners and others will therefore need to assess are the circumstances in which parents find themselves, rather than pie-in-the-sky surveys of aspirations, and maybe it is advisable to be wary of assumptions that are founded on this type of evidence. It is perhaps the task of practitioners to assess these and other assumptions that might prevail at the outset, and to help parents past them so that they can deal with their real-world circumstances.

For example, Burgess cites one case of a couple, Alex and Jason, who:

> were operating from the shared but unspoken assumption that a good mother not only copes but copes alone and that a father's place is on the fringe. . . . (This assumption) required Alex to keep control of every detail of her baby's life, although paradoxically she then felt put upon and completely out of control.[32]

It is worth noting that the assumption is shared in this case. As so often happens, the father himself may suffer from a real lack of confidence in his abilities as a parent, particularly with regard to young children (although he can acquire more of a stake later when the children are old enough to undertake joint activities or play). This situation is so often compounded by the father not being offered either information and advice, or the opportunity to spend time alone with his children in order to develop childcare skills of his own that will boost his confidence. But where does the mother's assumption come from? Is it partly derived from models of care from professionals that emphasise her role as the primary caretaker of her babies, who only asks for help from the father when, by inference, she cannot cope, and is thereby deemed to have failed when she does ask for such help?

With regard to simple *support* – a word that is often used in pregnancy – the picture is clearer, to the extent that it can be distinguished from involvement. Women value the support that they receive from their partners, and the supportive role that the latter play is important to them.[33] In total, 67% of pregnant women with a partner report receiving most support from him (80% of the men get most support from their partners; the difference here is largely one of maternal support – 11% of women get most support from their mothers, whereas only 2% of men get most support from their mothers).[34]

Is there an argument that mothers want support but not involvement? The social commentator Melanie Phillips has written that women will never let men look after children 'except as souped-up au pairs'.[35] This is to assert that they want support, but definitely not involvement by another autonomous parent. However, surveys do not test the one against the other. What is perhaps clear is that mothers can value support *and* involvement, but can *also* feel threatened if they perceive that their role as primary caretakers of their babies is being undermined. The element of threat will be emphasised by the premium that professionals put on the mother's role as primary caretaker of her children. It probably varies greatly for individuals and couples both from moment to moment, and as the children get older. From the viewpoint of the individual father, it may be difficult for him to know or second-guess where he stands in these circumstances, as he may be receiving some very mixed messages.

One example of this is found in Rebecca Abram's book *Three Shoes, One Sock and No Hairbrush*. Abrams takes a tough approach to fathers who, she claims, shirk their responsibilities. Yet on the other hand she does not want fathers to get too close, asserting that 'We categorically do not want fathers colonising the corner of our children's heart that is forever mummy's.'[36]

However, for health professionals, given that most fathers accept a supportive role in the antenatal period and that mothers value their partner's support, at the very minimum the need must be for the father's needs to be addressed to enable him to fulfil this role more effectively. Is it necessarily a bad thing if he gets involved in the longer term as a result?

Perhaps there is a straightforward conclusion to be drawn here – that the father will ultimately end up supporting the mother to the extent that he becomes involved. Perhaps that may be the price of continued support. If the father is to have a long-term role in the family, his role must become more than a contingent one. It must assume an autonomy where he develops skills and competences of his own – and the confidence as a parent that comes from acquiring them. It is that long-term engagement with the family that will ultimately support mothers the most. It is perhaps for practitioners to recognise that the father will probably be 'around' more consistently than their agency support to the mother can be.

Ultimately these are issues for parents to work out and decide between themselves, rather than for health professionals and practitioners to impose their own beliefs on parents. As suggested below, it is perhaps for health professionals and others to facilitate dialogue between the two parents. This will perhaps help them to anticipate such issues and help them to prepare for their parenthood together by acknowledging the father's potential as well as that of the mother. It is surely beneficial to the mother not to leave the task of unlocking the father's potential to her. It is equally important that the mother is not burdened with the suggestion that a good mother copes alone – a suggestion that is implicit in the father being ignored as a potentially equal partner in parenting and perhaps ultimately reinforced by suggestions that he has a supporter's role.

Men and mothers' networks: trespassers, guests or fellow parents?

- Neither mothers nor fathers can correctly be characterised as homogenous groups with regard to their expectations of each other – just as men and women generally can welcome, resist or be indifferent to either sex undertaking roles that are usually ascribed to the other.
- Service providers and project staff should be aware of the role played by service users in effectively determining who the service is used by (others who are comfortable with the group).
- This should be borne in mind when establishing 'parents' groups and programmes.

At the beginning of this chapter focusing on the value of fathers and engaged fatherhood, the attitudes of project workers and staff with regard to men and fathers were examined in the context of asking how to promote engaged fatherhood.

However, the experience of any service user can be affected as much by the attitude and welcome that he or she receives from other service users as by the attitude of workers and staff. Of course, the attitudes of workers and staff will have a bearing on the expectations of those service users for whom it is understood the service is intended, but it is likely that service users will also form their own understanding independently.

Fathers can experience a sense of exclusion from mothers when they seem to be trespassing on their social networks (e.g. when they bring their child to what may be called a 'mother-and-toddler group', even though there may be a headline policy that fathers are welcome to attend such a group).

A spokesperson for the charity Fathers Direct was discussing the need for fathers to establish 'father-and-toddler' drop-in groups to mitigate this exclusion on the BBC Radio 4 programme *You and Yours* on 29 June 2000 with a spokesperson from *Mother and Baby Magazine*. Her proposition was as follows.

> All the support networks that are set up for mums will continue to be there for scientific and biological reasons.

> This new role that dads want to take on, I applaud fully. But how long will it last when economics get back to full employment?

> There is a certain percentage of dads who want to be in the home and a certain percentage who do it because they can't find anything else to do.

> The network for new mothers is fantastic and will continue to be so. I have my doubts as to whether we will ever embrace dads into these groups. ... On a girls' night out you don't want a boy in there.

It is therefore necessary to draw a distinction between the support or involvement that mothers want from the fathers of their children in the home and the involvement that they want the father to undertake publicly. Mothers could be sensitive to charges of being unfeminine and unmotherly if it is their partner who is engaged in caring gestures towards the children in public – with the mother appearing to be cold and aloof – just as much as a father might hold back from such gestures for fear of being considered unmasculine.

Equally, other mothers like the impression given by the obviously engaged fatherhood of their partner, perhaps because this symbolises a modern and equal relationship or a cutting-edge appreciation of the value of fatherhood.

These are considerations that must be given weight when planning support programmes for parents. Whatever the ostensible purpose and client group of the programme, this can nonetheless be to some extent appropriated and revised by the attitudes and expectations of the service users themselves. This need not be conscious. If a 'new parent group' is in practice only attended by mothers, this can give rise to the belief that it is intended for their exclusive use. A father trespassing into this environment could encounter resistance unbeknownst to the programme worker. The tendency for the group to be attended only by mothers will thus be reinforced.

However, much as it is said elsewhere that men are not an homogenous group (e.g. when examining whether they are in some cases more or in other cases less comfortable about accessing services designed for men alone, or whether they prefer groups of both men and women), it has to be acknowledged that women are not an homogenous group either in exactly the same respects. On one level their view of fathers can also be to see them simply as other parents, who differ in style perhaps but not in value.

There may also be an interim position where mothers consider fathers to be welcome 'guests' of their networks. In effect this reserves the position that childcare – at least in public – is essentially understood to be the proper concern of mothers, but suspends such a position in the case of the individual father attending a group or undertaking any given activity (with the possible exception of one-on-one physical play, which is considered to be his proper domain and does not usually involve a group). The experience of a father in such a situation is a hybrid mixture of welcome and exclusion. This is probably the most common experience of all for public fatherhood.

The value to children of involved fathers

- Studies show that involved fathers can be valuable to children as attachment figures, and that they bring a range of benefits to the development of both boys and girls.
- Practitioners should therefore encourage involved fatherhood in the interests of children in the round, and not just as a narrow response to 'the problem with boys'.
- Fathers' capacity for involvement should not be perceived as competing with that of mothers, but as a resource for the family as a mutually supporting unit.

The Chief Executive of the NFPI, Mary MacLeod, has written that 'it does seem strange to decide to "make the case" for dads ... surely it should be self-evident that dads are a good thing – it certainly is to children.'[37] But again, often 'making the case' about the value that fathers bring to their children can be perceived to be at the expense of what mothers can bring. Indeed, the title of Mary MacLeod's paper was 'Ending the Fathers versus Mothers gender battle.' However, the essence of valuing what fathers can bring to their children is not to allege that mothers are deficient as parents (such that the input of the father is needed to make up for any such deficiency),[38] but rather to acknowledge that children benefit more from having two engaged and committed parents than from having one.[39]

It appears that it is this engagement and commitment, rather than an inherent value in his masculinity, which are the positive qualities that the father can bring to his children.[40] However, it also appears to be the case that the father's own interpretation of his gender role can often bring a different parenting style (e.g. leading the children in outdoor physical activity and play) which adds to the joint value of the couples' parenting. This is what is meant when it is said there is no 'magic' ingredient that fathers bring to parenting just by virtue of being male – they bring a style ingredient, rather than a substance ingredient that is valuable in itself. Moreover, the same applies to both parents. As Susan Golombok has stated about the kind of attachment that babies can form with involved fathers, 'it seems that there is nothing special about what mothers do with their babies'.[41]

Thus supporting fathers' involvement is not about threatening mothers by positing men's gender superiority as carers, nor about flattering men that their masculinity alone is of benefit to their children, but rather it is about supporting fathers as parenting team members in partnership with the mother. As has been said,[38] 'fathers and mothers behave in surprisingly similar ways'.

Differences in style may nevertheless exist, and often tend to arise when fathers are aware that they are being observed. This is due to a self-consciousness about behaving in public in ostensibly 'feminine' ways,[42] and also to a tendency to stand back from parenting gestures in 'feminine' spaces.[43]

There are also many specific indicators of the benefits of father involvement with children, which are summarised below.

1   According to Burgess, many of these benefits have been measured:

> Right through adolescence, and in many different ways, the benefits to children of positive and substantial father involvement can be measured: in self-control, self-esteem, life skills and social competence. Adolescents who have good relationships with their fathers take their responsibilities seriously, are more likely to do what their parents ask, and are less limited by traditional sex-role expectations. The boys have fewer behaviour problems in school, and the girls are more self-directed, cheerful and happy, and willing to try new things.[44]

2   Clare points out that the benefits are not just for boys:

> Tessman studied high-achieving women students from Massachusetts Institute of Technology. The typical father was described by his daughter as encouraging, stimulating, involving her in joint endeavours, showing trust in her growing abilities, and a playful and enjoyable companion.[45]

3   Clare also cites developmental benefits for children with engaged fathers:

> recent research strongly suggests that preschool children whose fathers are substantially engaged with and accessible to them (i.e. performing 40% of the care within the family) are more competent, more empathetic, more self-confident and less stereotyped in terms of gender roles.[46]

4   Clare also finds further evidence that involved fathers reduce gender stereotyping among their children:

> Most striking is the finding that a more actively involved father leads not to more but to less gender-role stereotyping behaviour in the children. That is to say, children and adolescents with positively involved fathers hold *less* traditional views as adolescents about gender stereotypes, dual-earner parents and about the parental sharing of childcare.[47]

5   Other studies show involved fatherhood reduces the likelihood of criminality in children:

> When fathers are involved with their children before the age of 11, the children are more likely to escape having a criminal record by the age of 21.[48]

It also seems that the father does not necessarily need to be resident for this effect to be achieved:

> Having a biological father who maintained a close relationship with his son, whether or not he lived in the family home, might be crucial in preventing susceptible boys becoming criminals.[49]

However, as is suggested above, this effect may be more marked among boys. The study by Buchanan and Flouri found that 'Children with involved fathers are less likely to be in trouble with the police', but noted that:

> Boys in particular are less likely to be in trouble with the police where they have 'involved' fathers. This relationship persisted even when we took into account several factors which are associated with adolescent delinquency.[50]

6   Golombok notes that children turn to involved fathers as attachment figures:

> The more fathers become involved with their infants, the more their infants are likely to seek comfort from them. ... This was demonstrated by Martha Cox and her colleagues, who investigated fathers' relationships with their babies, first when they were aged 3 months and again at 1 year old. The fathers who took delight in their 3-month-old infants, and who were affectionate and encouraging to them, were most likely to have securely attached 1-year-olds. It seems that there is nothing special about what mothers do with their babies. If fathers do the same, they too can have a close bond with their child.[51]

7   Golombok also found benefits in play and sociability among their peers for children with involved fathers:

> We have already seen from Martha Cox's research that men who spend time and enjoy being with their infants have a more secure relationship with them by the time they are a year old. Other studies have found the same. But it is not just the child's relationship with the father that is improved by the father's involvement; relationships with other children are better as well. In a study of preschoolers, those who were securely attached to their father at a year old were found to play more harmoniously with their peers.[52]

> When Lise Youngblade and Jay Belsky followed up children from age 3–5, they found that those who had a good relationship with their father at 3 years old had better friendships when they were 5.[53]

These children also show fewer behavioural problems:

> The National Survey of Families and Households, conducted in the United States, has shown that fathers who are actively involved

with their 5- to 8-year-old children have sons and daughters with fewer emotional and behavioural problems and who are more likely to get along well with others and do as their parents ask.[54]

In addition, they benefit from improved intellectual development:

> And it seems that it is not only children's social development that is improved by involvement with the father; children benefit intellectually as well. In a study that followed up 1-year-old children until the age of 7, those who had a positive relationship with their father were found to have higher IQ scores and do better when they entered school.[55]

8   Golombok concludes:

> The more that fathers are actively involved in parenting, the better the outcome for children's social and emotional development.[56]

9   An American Study conducted by Professor Howard Dubowitz has also reportedly found benefits both in self-esteem and in fewer symptoms of depression for children who live with their fathers. In addition, it has reportedly found that they have a greater sense of social acceptance. Professor Dubowitz has commented on his work in an interview with *The Sunday Times*:

> It clearly shows that a father's presence and involvement benefit the child. We need to find ways to encourage the positive and supportive roles of fathers and father figures in the lives of their children.
>
> Given all the permutations of what counts as family these days, when these kids describe having an adult male around, usually their biological father, they were doing better.[57]

The British study by Buchanan and Flouri also found that father involvement can reduce the incidence of mental health problems in later life for children in separated families. It is noted in Chapter 2 that there is currently much focus on the relationship between fathers and sons, but the principal beneficiaries here seem to be daughters:

> Involvement of the father or a father figure has a significantly protective role against psychological problems in adolescents in families where parents have separated. This finding is independent of whether mothers are also involved. The association between father involvement in adolescence and psychological distress in adult life is stronger for daughters than for sons. Therefore, early father involvement has an important protective role against both later psychological maladjustment in children whose parents have separated, and against adult psychological distress in women.[58]

10   In the UK, a recent Government initiative called 'Dads and Sons – a winning team' also seeks to capitalise on the benefits of fathers being engaged with their children's education.

Η However, this initiative has been criticised by some for not addressing fathers and daughters.

It is interesting that the study by Buchanan and Flouri cited above (which some news reports[59] anticipated in their coverage of the 'Dads and Sons' initiative) found that 'Father involvement at age 7 and mother involvement at age 7 significantly and independently predict higher educational attainment by age 20, and this applies to both girls and boys.[60]

References and notes

1   Kissman B (2001) *National Council of Voluntary Child Care Organisations. Are We Shutting Out Fathers? Conference Report*, p. 44.

2   Carvel J (2001) Big rise in support for unmarried parents. *Guardian*. **26 November**.

3   Warin J, Solomon Y and Lewis C (1999) *Fathers, Work and Family Life*. Joseph Rowntree Foundation, York.

4   Kissman B (2001) *National Council of Voluntary Child Care Organisations. Are We Shutting Out Fathers? Conference Report*, p. 5, citing Clough J et al. (2000) *Engaging Parenting in a Primary School Setting*. Children North East, Newcastle Upon Tyne.

5   Teen male suicides hit 'crisis' level; *BBC News Online (Health)*, 30 April 2001.

6   Hazel N, Ghate D and Shaw C (2000) *Briefing Paper for Policy Makers and Service Providers: fathers and family support services*. Policy Research Bureau, London, p. 2.

7   Warin J, Solomon Y and Lewis C (1999) Families as a whole underestimate the amount of childcare by fathers. In: J Warin et al. *Fathers, Work and Family Life*. Joseph Rowntree Foundation, York.

8   Clare A (2000) *On Men: masculinity in crisis*. Chatto & Windus, London, pp. 184–5.

9   Burgess A (1998) *Fatherhood Reclaimed*. Vermillion, London, p. 171.

10   Marin R (2000) At-home fathers step out to find they are not alone. *New York Times*. **2 January**.

11   Daycare Trust (2001) *Who Will Care? Recruiting the next generation of the childcare workforce*. Daycare Trust, London, p. 5.

12   Gingerbread (2001) *Becoming Visible: focus on lone fathers*. Gingerbread, London, p. 24.

13   Smithers R (2002) Schools are short of male staff, admits minister. *Guardian*. **8 January**.

14   Haughton E (2002) Men: your classroom needs you. *Independent*. **28 February**.

15   My italics.

16   Men wanted in primary schools; *BBC News Online (Education)*, 22 April 2002.

17   Cameron C, Moss P and Owen C (1999) *Men in the Nursery: gender and caring work*. Sage, London.

18   Daniel B and Taylor J (2001) *Engaging with Fathers: practice issues for health and social care*. Jessica Kingsley Publishers, London, p. 217.

19 *Nursery World*, 25 November 1999.
20 Cameron C (2000) What a difference a man makes. *Coordinate: J Natl Early Years Network.* **77**: 12–13.
21 *Nursery World*, 15 May 1997.
22 Daniel B and Taylor J, op cit., p. 215.
23 Warin J *et al.*, op. cit., p. 37.
24 Cowan CP (1988) Working with men becoming fathers: the impact of a couples group intervention. In: P Bronstein and CP Cowan (eds) *Fatherhood Today.* John Wiley & Sons, New York.
25 Carvel J (2001) Big rise in support for unmarried parents. *Guardian.* **26 November**.
26 Burgess A, op. cit., p. 178. See Ochiltree G (1994) *The Effects of Childcare on Young Children: 40 years of research.* Australian Institute of Family Studies, Melbourne.
27 See, for example, Roberts J (2001) The tiny feet that trample romance. *Independent.* **30 July**.
28 Warin J *et al.*, op. cit.
29 Clare A, op. cit., p. 184.
30 Watson WJ, Watson L, Wetzel W *et al.* (1995) Transition to parenthood. What about fathers? *Can Fam Physician.* **41**: 807–12. Citing Lamb ME, Pleck J and Levine J (1986) Effects of paternal involvement on fathers and mothers. In: C Lewis and M O'Brien (eds) *Reassessing Fatherhood.* Sage, Beverley Hills, CA, pp. 67–83.
31 Initial findings of the Families, Children and Childcare Project study launched during National Childminding Week in June 2002.
32 Burgess A, op. cit., pp. 132–3.
33 NCT Survey, *Becoming a Father*, by Singh D and Newburn M (2000), in association with Fathers Direct, National Childbirth Trust, London, pp. 39–40.
34 NCT Survey, op. cit., p. 41.
35 Phillips M (1999) A change in emphasis. *Sunday Times.* **30 May**.
36 Abrams R (2001) *Three Shoes, One Sock and No Hairbrush.* Cassell, London.
37 MacLeod M (2001) Ending the Fathers versus Mothers gender battle. In: *FatherFacts. Volume 1, Issue 1.* Fathers Direct, Newpin Fathers Support Centre, NFPI and Working With Men, London.
38 Burgess A, op. cit., p. 70. Couples parent in surprisingly similar ways. 'Of course, some fathers behave very differently from their wives, but in the land of averages – where most people dwell – there can be no doubt that, individually (as couples) and collectively (as gender groups), fathers and mothers behave in surprisingly similar ways. It is also the case that they do so in spheres where their behaviour has been thought to be particularly gender-oriented.'
39 Burgess A, op. cit., p. 183. 'One finding of particular interest to researchers has been that in two-parent households, children raised mainly by their fathers do better than those mainly raised by their mothers. Does this mean there is something innately superior about men's parenting? No. These children have *two* actively involved parents: their fathers as day-to-day caretakers, and their mothers devoting more time and energy to them after work than do most breadwinner fathers.'

40   A parent's gender is far less important in affecting child development than broader qualities such as warmth and kindness. From: What good are dads? In: *FatherFacts*, op. cit. For a review, see Burgess L, Clarke L and Cronin N (1997) *Fathers and Fatherhood in Britain*. Family Policy Studies Centre, London.

41   Golombok S (2000) *Parenting: what really counts?* Psychology Press, Hove, p. 19.

42   This can be drawn from the finding that they are more predisposed to engage in 'masculine' behaviours when watched. 'Researchers find that fathers engage in physical play more with sons than daughters, especially when there are other people around' (*FatherFacts*, op. cit., p. 6) and that 'Fathers are more inclined to hold their babies when mothers are not present' (*FatherFacts*, op. cit., p. 4).

43   Burgess A, op. cit., p. 97. 'Parenting styles are determined not by gender but by situation, and differences arise not through the amount of time fathers spend with their children, but the amount of time they spend *alone* with them and the degree of responsibility they hold for their daily routine. This realisation has alerted researchers to the possibility that many of the so-called gender differences between mothers and fathers may be situational in origin. It has been noticed that fathers are more likely to wipe their toddlers' faces in playgrounds or sports centres, where they feel they are in charge, than in supermarkets or restaurants, which they may see as female territory.' Citing Lewis C (1996) Fathers and preschoolers. In: ME Lamb (ed.) *The Role of the Father in Child Development* (3e). John Wiley & Sons, New York.

44   Burgess A, op. cit., p. 180. Citing Pleck JH (1996) Paternal involvement: levels, sources and consequences. In: ME Lamb (ed.) *The Role of the Father in Child Development* (3e). John Wiley & Sons, New York.

45   Clare A, op. cit., p. 177. Citing Tessman L (1982) A note of father's contribution to his daughter's way of loving and working. In: S Cath, AR Gurwitt and J Ross (eds) *Father and Child: development and clinical perspectives*. Little, Brown & Co, Boston, MA, pp. 2219–38.

46   Clare A, op. cit., p. 169. Citing Radin N (1994) Primary-caregiving fathers in intact families. In: AE Gottfried and AW Gottfried (eds) *Redefining Families: indications for children's development*. Plenum, New York, pp. 55–97.

47   Clare A, op. cit., p. 169. Citing Williams E, Radin E and Allegro T (1992) Sex role attitudes of adolescents raised primarily by their fathers. *Merrill Palmer Q.* **38**: 457–76.

48   What good are dads? In: *Fatherfacts*, op. cit., p. 7. Citing Lewis C, Newson J and Newson E (1982) Father participation through childhood and its relation to career aspiration and proto-delinquency. In: N Beail and J McGuire (eds) *Fathers: psychological perspectives*. Junction, London.

49   Hall S (2001) Crime linked to absent fathers. *Guardian*. **5 April**. This article reports research presented by clinical psychologist Jenny Taylor of the South London and Maudsley NHS Trust to the conference of the British Psychological Society, Division of Forensic Psychology, Birmingham, 4 April 2001.

50   Buchanan A and Flouri E (2001) *Father Involvement and Outcomes in Adolescence and Adulthood*. ESRC End of Award Report. Department of Social Policy and Social Work, Oxford University, Oxford, p. 2.

51   Golombok S, op. cit., p. 19. Citing Cox MJ, Owen MT, Henderson VK and Margand NA (1992) Prediction of infant–mother and infant–father attachment. *Dev Psychol.* **28**: 474–83.

52 Golombok S, op. cit., p. 22. Citing Suess G, Grossman K and Stroufe LA (1992) Effects of infant attachment to mother and father on quality of adaptation to preschool: from dynamic to individual organisation of self. *Int J Behav Dev.* **15**: 43–65.

53 Golombok S, op. cit., p. 22. Citing Youngblade LM and Belsky J (1992) Parent–child antecedents of 5-year-olds' close friendships: a longitudinal analysis. *Dev Psychol.* **28**: 700–13.

54 Golombok S, op. cit., p. 22. Citing Mosley J and Thomson E (1995) Fathering behaviour and child outcomes: the role of race and poverty. In: W Marsiglio (ed.) *Fatherhood: contemporary theory, research and social policy.* Sage, Thousand Oaks, CA, pp. 148–65.

55 Golombok S, op. cit., p. 22. Citing Gottfried AE, Gottfried AW and Bathurst K (1988) Maternal employment, family environment and children's development. In: AE Gottfried and AW Gottfried (eds) *Maternal Employment and Children's Development: longitudinal research.* Plenum, New York, pp. 11–58.

56 Golombok S, op. cit., p. 23.

57 Dobson R (2000) Children with father in family have a head start in life. *The Sunday Times.* **21 May**.

58 Buchanan A and Flouri E, op. cit., p. 2.

59 Fathers improve school results; *BBC News Online*, 28 February 2002.

60 Buchanan A and Flouri E, op. cit., p. 2.

CHAPTER 3

Facilitating involved fatherhood before and after the birth: principles

Do fathers want more involvement?

- Fathers seek involvement with their children, and patterns of care are changing.
- Fathers are increasingly open about their involvement with and attachment to their children.
- However, fathers underestimate and understate their own involvement, which can render their actual and potential involvement invisible to professionals.
- Fathers can be reluctant to make parenting gestures in public, and before professionals, thereby increasing this invisibility of their parenting.
- The period before and after the birth of children is perhaps the time when fathers are most visible and accessible for practitioners who are assisting father involvement.

The major factors influencing father involvement have been outlined as follows:

> The factors which most influence involvement are the dad's work hours and work preoccupations, his relationship with his partner, and his preparation for involved parenting.[1]

This shows the value of preparing fathers for parenthood around the time of the birth:

> Fathers who have participated in baby-care courses take on more care of their babies than fathers who have not. Such fathers keep closer to their babies, engage in more face-to-face interaction with them, smile at, look at, and talk to them more.[2]

However, perhaps the most visible measure of how fathers themselves are seeking some kind of involvement with their children today is the number attending their birth. A 1994 Royal College of Midwives survey showed 93% of new fathers both wanting and planning to be there.[3] In the recent National Childbirth Trust survey, *Becoming a Father*, 96% of the men had been with their partner during labour or the birth.[4]

Are these men just pressured to be there? Burgess points out that of the RCM respondents, 88% reported 'no pressure' to be there and 12% reported 'some pressure'.[5] However, whatever pressure was experienced by those who reported it, it would be unlikely to alter an intention to attend anyway – 93% of fathers both wanted and planned to be there.

Another highly visible measure of men seeking involvement is to be found in those less happy cases where men besiege the courts, or sometimes even the homes of judges, seeking enforcement of contact orders enabling them to maintain their relationships with their children after divorce.[6]

Another measure can be found by looking on bookshop shelves, where a spate of books on fatherhood can currently be found, ranging from self-help books to memories of strong father figures and anthologies of writing on fatherhood. Often referring to personal relationships, this large number of books seem to speak of fatherhood beginning to hold a publicly revealed appeal for men. Such publications have recently become so prevalent that they have been termed 'dadlit.'

Moreover, according to a Joseph Rowntree Foundation report published in April 2000, 'surveys show that fathers' involvement in the home has been increasing and that the "gender gap" in terms of average time spent caring for children has narrowed.'[7] The National Childbirth Trust survey, *Becoming a Father*, also reports that fathers are now more involved, stating that 'the role of men in relation to birth and parenting has changed dramatically over the last generation or so. Clearly men get a lot out of their closer emotional involvement in the pregnancy and life with a new baby.'[8] Burghes reports a fourfold increase in time spent on childcare by men since 1961,[9] representing a greater increase than for women. A study by the Equal Opportunities Commission, entitled *Working Fathers, Earning and Caring*, published in 2003 by Margaret O'Brien and Ian Shemilt, reported the finding that since the early 1960s relative measures of childcare by fathers and mothers showed continued growth in the relative proportion of parental childcare by fathers with children of all ages from about 12.5% to about 33.5%.

Although 'research also suggests that mothers in two-parent households still typically carry the major share of routine household responsibilities and of caring for children',[10] research has also found that fathers were the main carers for children in 36% of dual-earner families while mothers were working – more than any other individual.[11] And single-parent families are not always headed by a mother. In one in ten cases they are headed by a father – a position held by 179 000 men.[12] The 1999 Labour Force Survey counted 100 000 stay-at-home dads.[13]

Although many men are constrained to some extent by their own or others' identification of them as holding the breadwinner role, much recent publicity has also been given to some high-profile cases where fathers have reduced their working hours in order to spend more time with their families – a phrase which is now no longer a jibe. A very much larger number of fathers have expressed the wish to do the same, but do not hold positions where this is achievable.[14]

Fathers' involvement can often be understated and underestimated (often by the men themselves),[15] and fathers tend to hang back when in public or in the company of mothers.[16] Daniel and Taylor report a case study of the way in which fathers can hang back before professionals as well, thus masking their true level of involvement.[17] In the antenatal and postnatal periods, they are less likely to share their own concerns than are their partners'.[18] Even highly involved fathers lack an inter-male space to identify themselves to each other. Even when responding to surveys, they can be guarded: 'So controlled, unforthcoming and contained are most men that they are careful when completing surveys and questionnaires which, as a result, are difficult to interpret'.[19]

Thus identifying involved fatherhood can be difficult when men tend to regard it as a private activity. However, as the surveys mentioned above have found, it is more widespread than it may seem. It is perhaps only at its most visible and accessible in the antenatal and postnatal period.

'Yes, but only middle-class fathers are involved like that'

- There are urgent grounds for discarding the misconception that involved fatherhood is only about middle-class fathers.
- Working-class fathers caring for children, many in circumstances of disadvantage, are isolated and unsupported either by their communities or by professionals.

When 'making the case' for fathers' positive contribution to family life, many people are of the view that these are matters of concern only for a minority of (middle-class) fathers. It is therefore concluded that fatherhood is a marginal concern for those professionals and voluntary sector practitioners whose work is dedicated to mitigating the adverse effects of poverty and disadvantage.

Although it is not actually true that middle-class fathers are more involved with their children, there are reasons why this assumption is commonplace. Middle-class fathers are more likely to articulate their feelings for and their involvement with their children, and their involvement is therefore more apparent. They are also less likely to report difficulty with evolution in gender roles. It is not suggested that these expressions should not be taken at face value, but other factors should be taken into account before concluding that middle-class fathers are more involved than other fathers.

The assumption that middle-class fathers are more involved stems from the correct interpretation that there is more express social support and nominal acceptance for involved fatherhood in the middle class than elsewhere. However, the many competing concerns that often bear upon middle-class fathers in practice and tend to inhibit them from being as involved as they would like to be are commonly overlooked. Essentially these stem from the 'subscription fees' that are due for membership of the middle class (school fees, foreign holidays, cars and houses that have to be paid for). However, dropping out of the orbit of friends, family, loved ones and acquaintances is a heavy human price to pay for the salary cuts and career damage that it is feared will result from appearing not to be committed to work or pull one's weight in the workplace. It is feared that these perceptions (that often in fact occur in the minds of bosses and colleagues) will result from asking for time off work or a change in working hours or practices that would enable greater involvement with the family.

On the other hand, working-class fathers are less inclined to be articulate about their involvement with their children and families. This can have a deceptive effect, giving rise to the assumption that they are less involved. Again, there is a germ of truth here that leads to this assumption – but the truth is about why these fathers are less expressive about their involvement.

It is not a matter of lack of capacity to express feelings, involvement or emotions – perhaps due to educational disadvantage. Fathers who have suffered such disadvantage express all of these in practitioner workshops where they feel that they are permitted to do so and they are aware that their audience consists of professionals who support and value fatherhood. Those who have attended such workshops would absolutely reject the charge that in doing so they are playing to the gallery and saying what they think their audience wants to hear.

These fathers are less expressive about their involvement because they are aware of (as those who make the assumption that they are less involved are conscious of) the relative lack of express and nominal support for 'involved' fatherhood in their community as this term is understood in that community. This lack of express and nominal support is also the source of the resistance to evolution in gender roles in such a community that has already been mentioned.

However, the fact that there may be less nominal and express support for what practitioners might categorise as 'involved' fatherhood in working-class communities does not mean that it does not occur. It can occur in ways that are less apparent to middle-class professionals and commentators who are sometimes more apt to recognise and validate traditional family structures, and it can occur in ways that are accepted and understood in its own terms in that community.

Thus it is suggested that either involved fatherhood does occur in such communities in ways that the community understands in its own terms, but that outsiders are unable to recognise, or that involved fatherhood occurs in ways that the community does not tend to support.

If involved fatherhood does therefore occur in ways that are not understood by professionals or supported by the community, this makes the case for voluntary and statutory sector support by family support agencies and others to ensure that these involved fathers are not isolated within their community or marginalised by support agencies (as they are at present). Such isolation and marginalisation are themselves bound to increase the likelihood of adverse outcomes for children who are being cared for by isolated and unsupported fathers who are already in disadvantaged circumstances.

The third option to consider, of course, is that involved fatherhood does not in fact occur in working-class communities in ways that the community would endorse and understand, or otherwise. However, there are no grounds for such a blanket assertion. On the contrary, there is reason to believe that involved fatherhood does occur – and not as a matter of exception to the general rule – but that it does so in particular in ways that are not apparent to those who are used to middle-class employment structures. For example, commenting on how fathers can under-report their own involvement (another common factor contributing to the lack of awareness of involved fatherhood), James Levine, director of the Fatherhood Project at the Families and Work Institute in New York, said in an interview in the *New York Times* with specific reference to the concept of stay-at-home fatherhood:

The number of men at home taking care of their kids is the best-kept secret in American child care. Many of them, he said, are blue collar: 'cops and firemen working night shifts while their wives work days.' Such men are not unemployed and may not consider themselves stay-at-home fathers.[20]

In highlighting the relevance of involved fatherhood for working-class fathers, Daniel and Taylor report Clarke and Popay's findings that 'there are less class differences than might be anticipated, in that working-class men were as likely to seek "new fatherhood" as middle-class fathers were to be traditionalists.'[21] This reinforces the importance of not building assumptions about individuals on the basis of perceptions about their backgrounds.

Barriers to father involvement

* If practitioners sense a lack of involvement by a father, this may not reflect his own wishes but be attributable to external barriers to his involvement that are encountered by him.
* It may be appropriate for practitioners to explore these barriers with the father in order to facilitate his involvement.

In order to understand how fathers can become involved with their children, it is also necessary to look at factors which can tend to act as barriers to their involvement. A few have already been mentioned, but a list of factors is presented below. The first five were identified by Cowan and Cowan.[22]

1   Family role models are weak because most of the current generation of parents were raised primarily by their mothers.
2   Men have no models of male nurturers; women have strong feelings against abdicating their role as primary caretakers of their babies (this was also noted in the National Childbirth Trust survey, *Becoming a Father*: 'Just as many of the problems that women experience in motherhood stem from traditional attitudes to women's role in society, men may sometimes feel limited in their involvement in babycare because of cultural attitudes, often from women, which regard childcare as a predominantly female domain'[23]).
3   Most men do not feel as competent about caring for their babies as their partners do. Even a small amount of implicit criticism causes them to relinquish the role of caregiver.
4   Women who become full-time mothers might think that their role is threatened and the balance of matrimonial power has shifted if their partners become too active or skilled in childcare.
5   Men often find that they receive mixed or negative feedback from their own parents as they take on an active role in childcare. The cultural expectations that are placed on men by their families of origin have a major influence on the way in which they parent their children and how they share the task with their partners.
6   The UK has a culture of long working hours. Most of those who work more than 48 hours a week are men. One in four of them put in extra hours, and

one in ten work more than 55 hours a week.[24] Employers tend to perceive that only mothers are parents, a view which is reflected in the relative availability of maternity leave and paternity leave, although some men are exercising their right to unpaid parental leave (which mothers can claim as well as maternity leave).

7 Fathers are excluded from service delivery. A recent NFPI report found that 'very few services are specifically targeted at minority ethnic groups and fathers',[25] and fathers form a tiny percentage of the childcare workforce, so services are unaware of their needs and service environments become feminised. That is to say, men feel that they are trespassing in a space which they do not feel invited to enter. They see no images of themselves and no male staff (men represent 0.9% of nursery nurses, 1.5% of playgroup leaders, 3.3% of classroom assistants, 5% of playworkers, 3% of nursery teachers, 0.5% of childminders and only 17% of primary schoolteachers[26]). Even where men are taken into account as family members, this is increasingly only to assess whether they are inflicting domestic violence on their partners.[27]

8 Men's non-breadwinning parenting is typically assessed from a 'deficit' perspective – seeing fatherhood as a role that men generally perform inadequately.[28] When men are stereotyped as inadequate and even abusive parents, this stereotyping has a real adverse effect in demotivating fathers and male childcare workers and undermining their proper involvement with their children and those in their professional care.[29]

9 Men are excluded from information that would assist their parenting. Hospitals distribute information about babycare to the mothers on the wards, and the content is designed to be read only by the mother. Form 362 about the registration of a baby's birth is addressed only to the mother. Parenting books and websites have a discrete 'dad's section' but no 'mum's section', indicating fathers' secondary status as parents or that the word 'parent' has replaced the word 'mother' without incorporating the word 'father' as it once did. The National Childbirth Trust survey on fathers reported that 'Men generally felt that midwives, hospital doctors and GPs had made them feel welcome and included in discussions. But there was room for improvement. A third of men felt that health professionals talked only to their pregnant partner, rather than including them both in the discussion.'[30]

10 It must also be acknowledged that barriers exist within men themselves. The reluctance of some men to engage in any activity with remotely feminine associations, although often associated with peer group pressure and different private views,[31] can be deeply entrenched.

Supporting the 'supporters': information for fathers – and recognition?

- Men are admitted to the delivery room and to some service processes before the birth on the express or implied condition that their role is to support the mother.

> - Excluding the father from information that meets his needs cannot help him to fulfil this role, and fails to take into account the fact that women receive most support from their partners.
> - Furthermore, casting the father exclusively in a secondary 'supporter role' may suggest to mothers and fathers that fatherhood is a secondary, contingent condition of parenthood and that childcare is necessarily 'women's work'.
> - After the birth, the father's 'supporter role' is discarded completely, reinforcing this message. The father is not subsequently recognised as a parent, which will tend to undermine the support that he gives the mother.

As discussed above, at the very minimum the majority of mothers want some kind of support or 'involvement' from their partners. The term 'support' tends to be applied during pregnancy and the perinatal period. The concept of 'involvement' generally tends to be applied as a measure of the father's interaction with the growing family.

It is usually on the basis that men are there to support the mother that they are invited into the delivery room. And men understand that their partners need support during labour.[32] The fundamental assumption is that they are there to play a 'role' – in the sense of performing a specified function – and that the nature of this role is 'supportive'. In the Lavender study, 'All men agreed that their main role was "supportive"'.[33] By way of contrast, it is interesting to note that the mother is never described as playing a 'role'.

It being a given, apparently accepted by fathers, that the father is there to 'play a supportive role', two questions follow. First, is the father given enough information to play this role properly? And secondly, is the casting of the father in a merely supportive or secondary role (or even a 'role' at all) necessarily in the long-term interests of the mother?

On the release of the National Childbirth Trust survey, Belinda Phipps, Chief Executive of the NCT said:

> Fathers are important. This research shows that, contrary to common belief, most dads want to be involved right from the beginning. Yet it also demonstrates that many fathers, particularly young dads and those from ethnic minorities, are poorly informed and supported. Those responsible for helping new parents should help fathers be fully involved in pregnancy, birth and baby care. This survey shows men want and need more information.[34]

The survey found that fathers were poorly informed both before and after the birth:

1   A third of fathers felt left out of discussions (before the birth):

> A third of men felt that health professionals talked only to their pregnant partner rather than including them both in the discussion.[a]

---

[a] NCT Survey, p. ii

2   Men wanted more information after the birth:

> In the early days after the birth, the men wanted midwives to
> provide more information about what to expect from life with a
> new baby. At least one in three said they wanted more information
> about how to tell their baby is sick, how to cope with lack of sleep,
> and the role of fathers in the initial months of the baby's life.[a]

One of the two main reasons why men do not attend appointments is their uncertainty as to whether they are welcome or needed, so their lack of access to information in this instance is not necessarily attributable to a lack of either interest in attending appointments or opportunity to attend them during working hours. Men's uncertainty as to whether they are wanted or needed at appointments will, of course, be marked among the third who felt that they were excluded from discussions.

> The 448 men who had seen health professionals less often than they
> would have liked or had not attended any appointments gave a range
> of reasons for this. ... The most common were:
>
> > The timing of appointments was inconvenient or employers
> > wouldn't allow men time off work to attend ...
>
> Men were uncertain about whether they were welcome or needed.[b]

So where do men obtain their information if not from health professionals? It is perhaps unsurprising that they obtain most of the information from their partners. However, if their role is predicated as being a supportive one, it is questionable whether it is sensible or fair that the burden of informing the father should fall on the mother. Yet this is an inevitable consequence of excluding the father from the information loop.

However, the exclusion of the father from the information loop has more than just the short-term effect of burdening the mother during the pregnancy. It also serves to convey the impression that the business of childcare is 'women's work' and will thus tend to undermine the support that he gives the mother and his involvement as the child is reared.

As we saw in Burgess' case study of Alex and Jason, it was the joint expectation which the couple had formed that a good mother copes well *and alone* that led to the mother, Alex, feeling put upon and out of control. The sense Alex has of being put upon is clearly harmful to her relationship with Jason. But how had this joint expectation arisen? It is argued below that this expectation can, in practice, be suggested to parents by health professionals and service environments.

Undermining the support that the mother receives from the father clearly makes little sense for women when 'partners are the most heavily relied on support system for women during pregnancy.'[35] Yet where the mother perceives a lack of support from her partner this may well (as it did for Alex) have adverse consequences for their relationship. Moreover, tending to undermine the couple's relationship in this way makes little sense for women either, when the importance of a harmonious

---

[a] NCT Survey, p. v; [b] p. 9.

relationship between the parents cannot be overestimated, as is noted in *FatherFacts*: 'The ability to cope with the demands of a new baby depends on the quality of the relationship between mother and father. This is so for both men and women.'[36]

Not only is it not in the interests of women – risking impairing the parents' relationship also risks impairing the outcomes for children when, as Burgess points out, 'the single most important indicator of maladjustment in children is their parents' active hostility – to each other.'[37]

However, in this context, simple admonitions to the father to 'help' – which tend to imply that he should take his lead from and follow the instructions of the mother – may well be counter-productive in that they will tend to emphasise his secondary status as a parent, thereby *demotivating* him and inducing passivity in his parenting.

Recognition for fathers

Thus restricting the father to the role of supporter-at-best may be prejudicial to outcomes for the mother, the child and the whole family. However, taking this approach and addressing the issue in these terms is also an example of a contingent approach to evaluating the *father's* needs, as a parent or individual, whereby any such evaluation will tend only to be incidental to promotion of the interests of other family members. In maternity services, as they are indeed known, this contingent threshold is raised to the point of near-exclusivity by many services falling under directorates of women's health.

As has already been noted, when fathers are asked about being present in the delivery room, the issues centre on the 'role' that they might wish – or are expected – to play. Yet ask the mother what role she wants to play and the question appears absurd. She is there to perform an autonomous function – to give birth. Yet we do not think the question absurd in the case of the father.

The word 'role' when applied to the father's presence in the delivery room therefore predicates that he is not there to perform an autonomous function – he is there (using the dictionary definition of 'role playing') to 'perform a *specified* function'. Lavender's study, sympathetic to fathers' needs as it was, took it as a given that the father attends the birth on the basis of performing a role, and asked its respondents which role they intended to play.

Fundamental attitudes to the presence of fathers in the delivery room are revealed by analysing what is meant by the use of the words 'support' and 'role' as a measure of their presence. The inference is that becoming a father is not an autonomous function, but a social one. That is to say, it is specified by people – it is a 'role' that fathers 'play' rather than a position that they assume or a function that they execute by virtue of the fact of their child being born. Fathers, it might be supposed, should do as they are told.

Interestingly, Lavender corroborates the prevalence of this supposition by challenging it:

> Midwives should reject the view that the mother or midwife should define the role of the expectant father. Instead, she should emphasize the importance of a three-way team whereby decisions are made which are acceptable to all those involved.[38]

It therefore appears that health professionals may be effectively suggesting to parents that mothers moderate or 'gatekeep' the level of father involvement in their families by emphasising the father's 'role' as a 'supporter', suggesting that the father is only there to help so long as the mother requires that help, and failing to acknowledge him as one of the 'parenting duo'. Thus we have the joint expectation formed by both Alex and Jason.

So is fatherhood just a secondary, socially determined capacity of parenthood, whereby the father's proper function is only to help the mother? Few people would take this position, particularly when considering the child's perspective. To take just one example, the need to know who their natural father *is*, and the increasingly common search for their natural father by adopted children or those conceived by donor insemination, as a necessary component of their individual identity, tend to undermine the case that fatherhood is only a social function. These fathers, by their very absence, have played no social function in their children's lives. Indeed, they may well have been substituted by what are known as 'social fathers' (non-genetic fathers). It is therefore better, perhaps, for fatherhood to be understood as an autonomous function – as a *fact*. And if fatherhood is recognised as a fact, fathers must also be recognised on an autonomous basis, and their needs assessed and met as parents and individuals on a non-contingent basis.

As the NCT survey itself concluded:

> All maternity services should have an information and support strategy with clear objectives regarding fathers' information and support needs and identified ways of responding to them. The strategy should acknowledge that men have needs in their own right as parents and are usually the major supporters of women during pregnancy, in childbirth, and as they establish themselves as parents.[18]

However, at present the curtain comes down firmly on the father's role after the birth. He is assigned no role or function at all by health professionals, instead being dropped like a hot potato. All talk of being there to support his partner or otherwise is forgotten. He may well be smartly ushered out of hospital as soon as 'visiting' hours are over. The hospital medicalises the mother, who becomes a bed-bound patient recuperating with the baby on a ward. The father is demoted from 'supporter' to 'visitor' within moments of his child being born. The baby is tagged with the mother's name only. The birth-weight card features the mother's name, but not the father's. On discharge from hospital, the mother is given babycare information and products, but nothing is given to the father. Form 362 from the Registrar General concerning registration of the baby's birth is addressed exclusively to the mother, but it states that she 'may, perhaps' wish to discuss registration with the father.

Pregnancy is not just a medical condition, if it is one at all. It is a natural process whose effects do not end for the 'patient' – the mother – when she leaves hospital. It is a process that involves others, too – most significantly the newborn child and the father. Indeed, viewing pregnancy as a natural process has raised the question of whether births should necessarily take place in hospital at all. Perhaps the marginalisation of the father in the birth process is another (new) consequence of the medicalisation of the birth process – a process that sees the mother as a 'patient' and the father as another mere 'visitor' to the postnatal ward. Interestingly, the father is somewhat less subject to marginalisation if the birth takes place in his own home, for then it is the midwives rather than him who leave after the birth.

The precipitous fall in the father's status after a hospital birth goes hand in hand with a further decrease in the amount of information provided to him by health professionals. The National Childbirth Trust survey found that:

> Health professionals provided very little information on the social changes men might experience after the birth of their child. Midwives were reported as providing less information on the new father's role than on any of the other topics listed. Health visitors appeared not to provide much on this subject either. ... This suggests that despite the recommendations made by the Expert Maternity Group,[39] men may not always feel assured that support, information and expertise are readily available to them from health professionals in the early weeks following the birth.
>
>   These findings suggest that midwives and health visitors are not providing much of a service directly to new fathers.[a]

This finding is corroborated by Suzanne Speak in *Young Single Fathers: participation in fatherhood — barriers and bridges*:

> After the birth of the child there is even less potential for health services to support the fathers, other than at baby clinics, to which none of the men in this study had gone. The few father support groups which do exist attracted older divorced or separated fathers and had not been used by the fathers in this study.[40]

In these circumstances, the new father may well wonder whether the invitation for him to attend the birth was extended in entirely good faith. In the hospital his status has dropped from that of supporter to that of visitor within minutes, and his name is completely blanked from his baby's nametag. When the midwife or health visitor comes to visit the new mother and baby at home, he may well feel that he has no role to play at all, as little or no attention may be paid to his needs unless it is to answer a question he takes the initiative to put to the relevant professional.

The message the father receives from this change in status is a very mixed one — he now seems to have no status at all. Now that the baby is here, it seems as if it is women's work from now on as the visiting female health professionals pay exclusive attention to the mother and child.

When making an appointment, the phone rings and the health professionals do not ask if it is the father if a man answers. They may immediately ask for the mother, or they may say 'I'm coming to visit [mother's name]' or 'I'm the health visitor for [mother's name]'. Children's health records, including vaccination records, which they distribute to parents reassure the latter that 'Your details as the natural mother will only be disclosed to your family doctor and health visitor.' If the father's presence is acknowledged — no information about his employment, self-employment, parental leave or unemployment being ascertained — reference may be made to his 'going back to work'. At this time the mother, but not the father, may be sent a

---

[a] NCT Survey, p. 63

follow-up letter from the Hospital Liaison Midwife Service 'to give all women the opportunity to discuss experiences of pregnancy, labour and delivery'.[41]

The damage done to the father's involvement by this process of exclusion is potentially immense. Both the mother and the father are given to understand that it all falls to the mother from now on. However much the father came to learn about being a supporter at the birth, the stake he had *even in this secondary role* may well be undermined by his being so quickly discarded afterwards. Again, casual admonitions to the father to 'help'[42] – perhaps all he can expect at this time – only tend to reinforce his secondary status in both parents' eyes. After all, it is important that the mother knows what to do when the father 'goes back to work' and the natural order is seemingly restored.

As is further shown below in the section on the supporter role (*see* p. 74), the need is to meet the father's express requirement for more information and to recognise him as a parent in his own right.

Equally, it is also necessary to take the pressure off the mother by recognising that the exclusive focus on her immediate needs around the birth conveys the implicit message that she should bear all of the burden of parenting in the long term. Restricting the father to a merely 'supportive' role at this time ultimately reinforces the message that all childcare is 'women's work'. This must tend to severely damage and undermine the father's involvement, and may even have the ultimate effect that the mother ends up receiving *less* support from her partner.

It is therefore suggested that restricting the father to the role of supporter, even where services equip him adequately for this role, fails ultimately to meet the needs of both parents, and fails even the contingent test of meeting the needs of mothers.

Breastfeeding and cot death: campaigns that already address fathers

* These two health promotion campaigns recognise that mothers and fathers are joined in a relationship, even though the campaigns address fathers in order to meet the needs of mothers and children.
* These campaigns set precedents for recognising that the needs of mothers and fathers are not wholly gender distinct – they also both become parents in the context of existing relationships.
* Mothers and fathers should be helped in their own dialogue as parents, rather than being divided by traditional gender role expectations.

Breastfeeding

If any ordinary person was to be asked about the attributes of mothers and fathers that qualify them for childcare and rearing children, one of the first attributes that would be assigned to the mother would be her ability to breastfeed. Breastfeeding might therefore be considered to be one area above all where health professionals should target information and support exclusively at the mother.

However, campaigners promoting breastfeeding have more recently become aware of the benefits of addressing fathers in their promotional message. Launching a poster campaign to promote breastfeeding in 2000, Public Health Minister Yvette Cooper stated that 'For a long time we have assumed that breastfeeding has nothing to do with men. We know that women who are most likely to start breastfeeding say that they have support from male partners.'[43]

The La Leche League also distributes a leaflet entitled *The Breastfeeding Father* which explains the importance of the father for successful breastfeeding. In addition, the National Childbirth Trust explains how fathers can make a difference, noting on its website:

> One important contribution that you can make as a father surprisingly concerns breastfeeding. The father's approval of a partner's breastfeeding has been identified as a key factor in their partner's decision to do so and its subsequent success.[44]

Important as breastfeeding is for the mother and her child, acknowledging the benefits of targeting men with information about breastfeeding is essentially founded on a more fundamental recognition – that parents have a relationship not only with their newborn child but also with each other.

Ignoring this relationship does not merely result in loss of the opportunity to unlock the father's potential as an involved parent or his specific support for breastfeeding. As the Cowans' research (*see* p. 33) into preparing couples for parenthood appears to show, the couples with prepared fathers experienced radically less relationship breakdown – selective preparation for parenthood actually has an effect in undermining the relationship between parents.

Ignoring the couple's relationship must increase the likelihood that the experience of having a newborn baby in the home will come between the parents, rather than uniting them in a joint project.

Recognition of the relationship between the parents, such as is found in the campaign to promote breastfeeding, therefore argues against the selective provision of information and support to just one member of that relationship. It argues for the provision of information and support for *both* parents in the interests of promoting a mutually supportive parenting partnership and the facilitation of a joint dialogue about the couple's expectations of parenthood.

Cot death

Another example of health professionals beginning to address men directly, albeit only contingently in seeking to promote child health, is provided by the campaign against cot death. A *BBC News Online* article about the campaign reported that:

> The Foundation for the Study of Infant Deaths (FSID) believes the emphasis should shift towards men because the message is not getting through. The organisation is targeting men to make them aware of the risks of smoking near very young babies. Joyce Epstein from FSID said: 'The mother–baby relationship is the one which gets the most attention and there tends to be a lack of awareness of the effect of things that dads do in relation to their baby's health.'[45]

> A study by the Imperial Cancer Research Fund has since found that parents can undermine *each other's* resolve when attempting to quit smoking during pregnancy.[46]

This campaign thus also provides a specific example of the importance of recognising the significance of the relationship between the parents, and not just the mother–child or father–child relationship.

These are further grounds for the need (argued for later in this book) for health professionals to facilitate a dialogue between the parents in order for them to form *their own* joint expectation of their parenting that will meet *both* their needs.

References and notes

1   *Fatherfacts, Volume 1, Issue 1* (2001) Fathers Direct, Newpin Fathers Support Centre, NFPI and Working With Men, London, p. 4 with footnote.
2   *Fatherfacts*, op. cit., p. 3 with footnote.
3   Royal College of Midwives (1994) *Men at Birth Survey*. Royal College of Midwives, London.
4   Around 90% of the men were present during both labour and the birth, 4% were present only during labour and 6% were present for the birth but not throughout labour. National Childbirth Trust (2000) *Becoming a Father*. National Childbirth Trust, London, p. 49.
5   Burgess A (1998) *Fatherhood Reclaimed*. Vermillion, London, p. 123.
6   Dyer C (2001) Fathers picket judges over child access. *Guardian*. **30 October**.
7   Joseph Rowntree Foundation (2000) *A Man's Place in the Home: fathers and families in the UK*. Joseph Rowntree Foundation, York, p. 3.
8   NCT Survey, *Becoming a Father*, by Singh D and Newburn M (2000), in association with Fathers Direct, National Childbirth Trust, London, p. 43.
9   Burghes L, Clarke L and Cronin N (1997) *Fathers and Fatherhood in Britain*. Family Policy Studies Centre, London.
10 Joseph Rowntree Foundation, op. cit., p. 3.
11 Joseph Rowntree Foundation, op. cit., p. 3.
12 Gingerbread (2001) *Becoming Visible: focus on lone fathers*. Gingerbread, London, p. 5.
13 Office of National Statistics (1999) *Labour Force Survey*. ONS, London.
14 See, for example, 'Time to quit for the family'; *BBC News Online (Business)*, 22 January 2002.
15 Warin J, Solomon Y and Lewis C (1999) *Fathers, Work and Family Life*. Joseph Rowntree Foundation, York.
16 Burgess A, op. cit., p. 85.
17 Daniel B and Taylor J (2001) *Engaging with Fathers: practice issues for health and social care*. Jessica Kingsley Publishers, London, p. 50.
18 NCT Survey, op. cit., p. iv.
19 Clare A (2000) *On Men: masculinity in crisis*. Chatto and Windus, London, p. 77.
20 Marin R (2000) At-home fathers step out to find they are not alone. *New York Times*. **2 January**.
21 Daniel B and Taylor J, op. cit., p. 137.
22 Cited in Watson WJ, Watson L, Wetzel W *et al.* (1995) Transition to parenthood. What about fathers? *Can Fam Physician*. **41**: 807–12.
23 NCT Survey, op. cit., p. 74.
24 Ward L (2002) UK still a nation of workaholics. On the TUC report *About Time. Guardian*. **4 February**.

25 NFPI (2001) *National Mapping of Family Services in England and Wales: a consultation document.* NFPI, London.

26 Daycare Trust (2001) *Who Will Care?* Daycare Trust, London, p. 5.

27 Morrod D (2000) Brief encounters – picking up signals of relationship distress. *Pract Midwife.* **3**: 27–9.

28 Hawkins AJ and Dollahite DC (1997) *Generative Fathering: beyond deficit perspectives.* Sage, Thousand Oaks, CA.

29 Gingerbread (2001) *Becoming Visible: focus on lone fathers.* Gingerbread, London, p. 24. Daycare Trust, op. cit., p. 5. Clare A, op. cit., pp. 184–5.

30 NCT Survey, op. cit., p. ii.

31 Williamson H (1998) *Boys, Young Men and Fathers. Ministerial Seminar Report.* Home Office Voluntary and Community Unit, London.

32 NCT Survey, op. cit., p. 50, citing Lavender T (1997) Can midwives respond to the needs of fathers? *Br J Midwifery.* **5**: 92–6.

33 Lavender T (1997) Can midwives respond to the needs of fathers? *Br J Midwifery.* **5**: 92–6.

34 Fathers Direct and National Childbirth Trust press release, *Government-funded Study of 'Blair Fathers' Demands Better Support for New Dads,* 11 September 2000.

35 NCT Survey, op. cit., p. 1. See also Kroelinger CD and Oths KS (2000) Partner support and pregnancy wantedness. *Birth.* **27**: 112–19.

36 *Fatherfacts,* op. cit., p. 4 with footnote. See, for example, Berman P and Pedersen F (eds) (1987) *Men's Transition to Parenthood.* Lawrence Erlbaum, Hillsdale, NJ.

37 Burgess A, op. cit., p. 178. See Ochiltree G (1994) *The Effects of Childcare on Young Children: 40 years of research.* Australian Institute of Family Studies, Melbourne.

38 Lavender T, op. cit., p. 95.

39 Expert Maternity Group (1993) *Changing Childbirth. Part 1. Report of the Expert Maternity Group.* HMSO, London.

40 Speak S (1997) *Young Single Fathers: participation in fatherhood – barriers and bridges.* Family Policy Studies Centre, London.

41 The author encountered all of these in 2001, after the birth of his and his partner's second child, except in the first telephone call from the health visitor who said 'Hello, I'm the health visitor for the family and the new baby. Can I speak to [mother's name]?'. When she arrived she spoke into the entryphone, introducing herself as 'the health visitor for [mother's name]'. All midwife appointments were made as described when the author (who works from home) answered the telephone.

42 This was also experienced by the author in the delivery room, after the birth, but not during the home visits. In general, however, as in 1995, the atmosphere was positive and inclusive despite the tension of the birth. At antenatal appointments the picture was more mixed.

43 Breastfeeding campaign targets men; *BBC News Online,* 15 May 2000.

44 nctpregnancyandbabycare.com. Becoming a dad – what to expect; 15 February 2002.

45 Fathers urged to quit smoking; *BBC News Online,* 9 June 2001.

46 Men wreck smoke-free pregnancy; *BBC News Online,* 21 November 2001.

CHAPTER 4

Reaching fathers: assessing needs, and methods

The previous chapter examined the 'supporter' role assigned to fathers, apparently with their acceptance. However, it was also noted that this 'role' is one that may be heavily scripted for them, and indeed that the term 'role' itself predicates a specified function that fathers are under a degree of compulsion to adopt.

The supporter role assigned to fathers was contrasted with the maternal function of giving birth – which is never described in terms of 'playing a role', for reasons that are somewhat more self-evident. It was argued that confining men to a supporter role is not necessarily in the interests either of mothers or of the long-term relationship between parents.

Fathers' needs as parents in their own right need to be looked at more closely. For example, do fathers, subscribe to the 'supporter' role because they feel it is only on this basis that they are invited to be involved in their partner's pregnancy? And what do they feel about another word that is often associated with fatherhood, namely responsibility?

However, it is also important not to overlook the needs and issues that bear upon individual men which stem from their perceptions of what their masculinity involves. Perceptions that are held by others about what masculinity means will also bear upon individual men both directly and indirectly. In recognising issues of masculinity and the needs of individual men, care must be taken to distinguish between men's public and private lives, where different aspects of maleness may prevail. Services that are designed to meet the needs of individual men may need to be sensitive to the distinctions between the public and private father.

The roots of men's exclusion from services

- In working with families, and in health services, men are often described as 'hard to reach'.
- However, services that concentrate on the mother as the access point to the family often exclude fathers either *ab initio* or by process.
- It is for services to address the roots of men's reluctance to seek support, or to circumvent this reluctance by appropriate interventions, rather than to collude with it in the interests of supporting men and their families.

In assessing fathers' own needs, the question arises as to whether fathers are themselves reluctant to attend to their own needs, and whether they are sometimes more comfortable about subscribing to the supporter role because this role posits the priority of their partner's needs.

If it is the case that fathers are suppressing their own needs because of a reluctance to admit them, or because they feel uncomfortable about addressing them, this reluctance and discomfort need to be examined and understood if the needs of fathers are to be attended to successfully and appropriately.

Men's reluctance to address their own needs often leads to their being described as 'hard to reach'. This description itself then often leads to inertia in attending to men's needs, rather than an examination of the roots and causes of this reluctance and how these may be circumvented and those needs met. The assumption is usually made that the roots and causes of men's reluctance to address their own needs lie within them and not in external factors associated with the delivery of services. Put crudely, it is often felt that if they are excluded at all (and it is seldom conceded they are), this is only because it is their fault anyway. This defensive attitude is then often reinforced or informed by negative assumptions and stereotypes about men.[1]

Men can also be subject to a cumulative process of exclusion from services that they do attend or in which they are initially involved. Williams refers to informal models of intervention that may be operated by health visitors that are mother focused or mother-and-child focused that 'lead to a focus upon women as gatekeepers to families, and also confirms and reinforces women's caring responsibilities within the home.'[2] This is also an interesting commentary on the effects of casting men in the supporter role.

Daniel and Taylor report Edwards' 1998 study of practitioners who:

> emphasized the importance of engaging with men, [but] when observed in practice they reinforced traditional messages that childcare is women's work and they regularly missed any opportunity to engage with the men they did encounter.[3]

This process of exclusion has also been noted earlier, when it was observed that men's uncertainty about whether they are wanted or needed at antenatal appointments, and their subsequent non-attendance, will be marked among those who felt that they were excluded from discussions which they had already attended (*see* p. 54).

The processes of exclusion also begin early. An Ofsted report in 2002 into Sex and Relationships Education (SRE) in schools observed that 'Boys feel that this support and advice is often aimed only at girls. While not necessarily true, the perception discourages them from seeking help.'[4] The report also recommended that more advice should be made available to young parents of school age, especially fathers.

As a further example, Brunt notes that although at the registration stage in the child protection process 65% of natural fathers and 25% of stepfathers are mentioned as playing a significant part in the child's life, 'professionals do not routinely examine *how* these men are significant in their children's lives, and whether their involvement in subsequent planning would be of benefit.'[5]

Absurdly, professionals' preconceptions about childcare being the exclusive role of women run so deep, the marginalisation of the father is so ingrained in these processes, and possibly assumptions about his abusiveness are also being taken as such a given,[6] that 'child protection investigations tend to focus on mothers, whether they are the alleged perpetrators or not.'[7] As Daniel and Taylor further point out, citing Dempster, 'Even in cases of sexual abuse, the work tends to concentrate on the mother's ability to protect the child from further abuse.'[8]

What is ridiculous here is that notwithstanding stereotypes of abusive masculinity that adversely inform many ordinary people's and professionals' attitudes about men's involvement with children in many varied contexts, Daniel and Taylor also conclude that when it comes to protecting children the marginalisation of the father even in this of all contexts is so acute that 'The potential risk that fathers and other male figures may pose both to children and women tends to be minimised in child protection.' By the same token, it goes almost without saying that they also conclude 'The potential for a father to be an asset to his child is consistently overlooked within child care and protection practice.'[9]

The need for a positively grounded awareness of masculinity

> • When working with fathers, a fundamental acknowledgement of the positive value that they can bring to their children and families is essential.
> • This acknowledgement is best informed by an awareness of issues pertaining to individual men's appreciation of masculinity.

It was acknowledged earlier in the examination of barriers to father involvement that barriers to their involvement in parenting and with their children exist within men themselves. Nonetheless, these internal barriers – allied with peer group or family pressures, for example – often coexist with conflicting private views and a personal wish to be involved.

It is essential to an understanding of the desire of fathers to be involved with their children, just as it is to an understanding of the roots of their reluctance to address their own needs and seek support, to have a properly informed appreciation of the issues relating to their own masculinity that can act as either barriers or facilitating factors in both areas.

There is currently little awareness of these issues, or of how they bear upon men, informing service provision. This lack of awareness represents a significant external factor preventing men and fathers from being prompted or encouraged to address their own needs and from using services. Where exclusion of men is acknowledged, as in the NFPI service mapping, uncertainty exists as to whether existing services should be made more accessible to men, or whether new services should be designed that are specifically targeted at them.

However, Lloyd makes the further point that before lack of appreciation by health professionals and others of issues pertaining to masculinity affecting men's take-up of services ('blame the professional') is used as a substitute for blaming the fathers for being 'feckless and irresponsible', 'we also have to recognise ... that men are generally reluctant users of services, especially support services.'[10] Williams also observes that 'The exclusion reported by many fathers from assessment and care delivery is compounded by fathers' own feelings, thinking and actions.'[11]

Yet hard as men may be to reach in this respect, it will be all the harder if the message conveyed to them is that they are failing and that because of this their behaviour needs to be corrected. It is unlikely that this is a message that men want to hear or that will lead to positive change. It is much more likely to lead to men withdrawing even further.

Views about masculinity that are held by others affect men's behaviour

> • Individual men's appreciation of masculinity is influenced by internal and external factors, by what they want as individuals, and by what is permissible for men and for fathers.
> • Messages that include positive suggestions about what is permissible and valuable behaviour may carry more weight than exclusively negative messages that indicate what is prohibited.
> • Men's behaviour changes when changes occur in the wider context of societal attitudes and choice is available.
> • Messages seeking a change in men's behaviour need to address societal attitudes and not men exclusively.

Societal perceptions about behaviour that is deemed to be masculine (including both positively and negatively viewed behaviours) that are held by others as much as by individual men themselves may also act to inhibit individual fathers' involvement with their children and, by extension, their use of services designed to support their parenting. Peer group pressure has already been noted as a factor that influences behaviour. By the same token, such pressures and perceptions about what constitutes masculine behaviour may act to encourage participation in positively viewed behaviours such as engaging in outdoor play and activities.

In other words, internal barriers or facilitating factors that influence men's involvement with their children may often initially arise from direct external pressure or from their second-guessing societal views about behaviours that they perceive will be approved of or disapproved of, rather than arising from a core gender identity.

Barriers like these which stem from outside, as opposed to those which stem from attitudes that an individual may hold autonomously, are relatively easily lowered when changes in societal attitudes occur. This process is facilitated when men are allowed to make choices previously denied them, such as attending the birth of their children,[12] or taking paternity leave now that companies have been offering it. Factors that facilitate men's involvement will also be given greater impetus by positive messages showing men how to 'get it right'. For one thing, they have probably already heard about what men are doing wrong.

Change as a positive choice by men

> - Messages that value positive behaviour by men may be more effective than exclusively negative messages indicating what is prohibited, as they enhance rather than undermine self-esteem in men.
> - Men's behaviour changes when changes occur in the wider context of societal attitudes and choice is available as much as it does by engineering change from within.

Interestingly, it is often said that 'men are changing', but the way in which this change occurs is less often examined. However, Williams citing the work of Connell, admits both change and the exercise of choice by men themselves:

> Perhaps the most important issue for practitioners, managers and policy makers within Connell's work is that there is evidence that masculine identities are not fixed, that men's identities are changing, and that men can make choices about status, power, parenting and health. Evidence here suggests, for example, that individual men (particularly the African–Caribbean and white fathers here) were involved in temporary or permanent roles as the main carer for children, and some outlined shared care for children with their partners/wives.[13]

Incidentally, it is the exercise of choice by men themselves that is the key to the value of providing positive role models for men and fathers as much as it is to that of the corrective–coercive messages aimed at the male-as-perpetrator which have predominated in recent years. Moreover, emphasising positive role models has the benefit of building rather than undermining men's confidence about the value that they are perceived to bring to their children and families – as well as to society as a whole.

In this context it is equally important to provide practical opportunities for men to exercise choice to effect change in their behaviour. Having been provided with the opportunity to attend the birth, nine out of ten fathers now do so. As well as role models, men need to be offered choice as individuals.

For example, few men are in a position as far as their employment is concerned, to work more family-friendly hours, although much attention has recently been paid to a few who have had the bargaining power to adjust their contracts.

Implications for service design: something about football?

> - Positive messages and choices should not be determined by stereotypical gender assumptions as narrow as negative men-as-perpetrator messages. The father-as-playmate model should not be overemphasised at the cost of other types of involvement.

- Not all men like football (as assumed by many football-themed service models).
- The association between fathers, sons and football should not obscure or act to prejudice the positive relationships that men have with their daughters, nor should it impose expectations that men should treat their sons and daughters differently.

It seems that services which address fathers' needs sensitively have to combine two elements. First, they must focus on actions and activities that tend to appeal to them *as men*,[14] taking into account their needs as individuals, but also as individuals who are subject to societal views about what is permissible behaviour for men. Secondly, they must be informed by a fundamentally positive view of men,[15] thereby building rather than undermining confidence about their perceived value as family members.

It should be emphasised that the designing of services to appeal to men must not ignore individual needs. For example, although many men like football, not all do, and using football as a medium or peg for services, or footballers as role models, will not exercise a universal appeal (e.g. the *Dads and Sons: a winning team* pamphlet features well-known footballers and offers tickets to the FA Cup).

Although football is the most popular team sport played by men, walking (48%), snooker (18%), cycling (15%) and swimming (13%) were more popular than football (10%) among the 80% of men who engaged in at least moderate physical activity according to a survey by the Office of National Statistics in its *Social Focus on Men*.[16] It is also said that more men go fishing than attend football matches every Saturday.

Although many men do take their children to football matches (both boys and girls), care should be taken when emphasising the relationship between fathers and sons that it is not seen to imply by default that relationships between fathers and their daughters are somehow inherently problematic and too sensitive an issue to approach, or simply not worth supporting.

This emphasis has tended to come about as the 'problem with boys' has moved up the political agenda. More recently it has been argued that problem behaviours exist among girls and that these should also be recognised in service provision, from which it is argued they are excluded by the emphasis on difficult behaviours and poor outcomes which affect boys.

It has been found that fathers express intimacy through shared activities with children, such as watching television and shared sporting or leisure activities and that these provide excellent opportunities for general conversation.[17]

However, before too much emphasis is put on fathers playing football with their sons, sensitivity should also be exercised in not boxing men into public expectations of masculinity that do not sustain the variety and complexity of the nature of their relationships with their children.

Lewis notes that fathers 'engage in physical play more with sons than [with] daughters, especially when there are other people around.'[18] It may be noted that this effect may now well be on the increase in the UK as physical contact between men and children (particularly girls) in public, has become viewed as problematic.

Lewis goes on to cast doubt on the overall differences in men's treatment of their sons and daughters:

> large-scale reviews and meta-analyses … do not support the assumption that men treat their sons and daughters differently. The few studies which show a difference may simply reveal an expectation about how men should treat their children rather than a clear influence on the child's sex-role development.[19]

It is therefore important that service design should not be driven by single-model expectations of masculinity if it is both to reflect the reality of the lives of fathers and children and to benefit individual men's engagement with their daughters as well as their sons.

Working assumptions of men's health projects: examples

- An analysis of working assumptions about young men shows by way of a variety of examples how young men and fathers can be supported by programmes that take barriers to constructive behaviour into account, rather than adopting a uniquely corrective or prescriptive approach.
- The working assumptions of these programmes provide further examples of barriers to involvement with their families and with support programmes that are encountered by young men.

Further important work by Trefor Lloyd about the experience of projects currently targeting services at men specifically includes a report on projects working in the field of young men's health, written with Neil Davidson.[20]

Reporting on a variety of aspects of their projects, among those covered are the projects' main working assumptions with regard to young men. A number of **major issues** for services specifically targeted at young men are revealed in these guiding assumptions, including the way in which men 'slip through the net and disappear' in traditionally modeled services. In Lloyd and Davidson's book the Coventry project entitled *Supporting Young Dads* reported that:

1 **Men slip through the net and disappear with traditional service models.** 'Recognised that with Government initiatives to combat teenage pregnancy, young men need to be included in service provision as so much existing provision is aimed at young women. Existing approaches to young men do not work, and they easily slip through the net and disappear …'

Other important factors mentioned in the paragraphs above are identified by other projects. For example, the *Cornwall Young Fathers Group* reported exclusion, like many projects, but also noted the effects of the bad press that they receive:

2 **A bad press affects young men's self-esteem.** 'Young fathers lack services targeted at them and do not access mainstream services.

Young men may need support in order to take full responsibility for their children. Young men receive a "bad press" which affects their self-esteem.'

The *Young Men's Health Promotion Roadshow* noted the absence of male staff in service environments and concluded that this reinforces the belief that their work is therefore an issue for women only.

3   **An absence of male staff defines services as 'women's work'.**
'Young men have a problem with taking responsibility for health issues and consequently are negligent of their own health. Health issues (e.g. in school) are stereotypically dealt with by women workers, reinforcing a message that health is a "women's issue" ...'

Other projects noted the effects of masculine discourses and the existence of different private views:

4   **Men have difficulties communicating where there is no masculine template for the discussion, and this tends to make them invisible as caring parents. They often have different private views (and behaviours) to those they express when subject to peer group pressure.**

Young men do not have or allow themselves a safe 'space' in which they can share how they feel. (Young People's Health Project, Birmingham)

The aim is to bring out young men's hidden caring side. They need to learn to communicate and find alternatives to the stereotypes.
(Wiseguys Project, Manchester)

It is recognised that young men suffer from peer pressure to conform to ideals of masculinity. Young men often behave very differently individually to how they are in group settings, where they feel compelled to play up to stereotypes.
(42nd Street, Manchester)

The importance of role models, masculinity and the problems presented by health workers' assumptions about men were noted by other projects:

5   **Role models are important for men, and masculinity is an underlying issue, sometimes problematically so for health workers.**

... young men need role models. There has been no specific focus on masculinity, but this has arisen as a training/consultancy need as the work has developed. (Community Responses to Persistent Young Offenders, Wolverhampton)

That young men have difficulties in asking for help, and lack communication skills. That workers often have difficulties with young men's attitudes and behaviours and with their own assumptions.
(Loudmouth Educational Theatre Company, Birmingham)

In general it is noteworthy that the projects are almost always founded on an essentially sympathetic and understanding set of assumptions about men, taking into account those areas where they need support.

Assessing men's needs around the time of the birth

- When practitioners attempt to meet men's needs, those needs may be obscured by men's assumption of the supporter role.
- The scripting of the supporter role by health professionals themselves may also act suggestively on both parents, tending to promote gatekeeping by mothers and undermining men's confidence as parents.
- Men may feel obliged to accept the supporter role as permitting entry into a female environment, and suppress their own needs which that environment does not encourage them to express.
- Mothers may act to indemnify the father's masculinity by giving him permission to engage in childcare. Scripting the supporter role for men may inhibit the operation of this indemnity.
- Practitioners need to take men into account as parents in their own right, not just as supporters.

A question that was raised earlier concerns what men feel about the supporter role – a role which it is suggested is heavily prescribed for them. However, the fact of it being prescribed does not rule out the possibility that the men nonetheless voluntarily assume this role and would continue to assume it even if they were offered other choices.

One suggested reason why they might be inclined to do this is that the supporter role posits the priority of their partner's needs, and men might subscribe to the supporter role because they are reluctant to address their own needs, or because they do not agree with the suggestion that they have any needs of their own.

Burgess suggests that men can act as 'agents of their own exclusion' for reasons often associated with views about real men being pillars of strength:

> The antithesis of male control is Nappyland, where tantrums rage and edicts are constantly ignored, a club which few boys dare join if they value their heterosexuality. For the milky world of mother-and-child represents, in our culture, the very essence of femininity ... the fear of being branded 'not man enough' continues to make men agents of their own exclusion, and drives a wedge between them and the development of skills necessary to be an active father.[21]

However, it is also argued here that men might feel that assuming the supporter role is a condition of their invitation and entry into what they perceive as a female domain (the 'milky world of mother and child'), which they are obliged to accept. Watson and Watson suggest that conditions can be imposed by mothers and reinforced by health professionals:

An important factor for an expectant father's self-recognition and accept-ance of his parenthood is his partner's view of him as an active participant in the pregnancy, a view that can be reinforced by a family physician.[22]

The impact of health professionals' attitudes was also noted in the National Child-birth Trust survey, lending weight to the suggestion that the supporter role is heavily scripted for men but may not reflect all of his needs:

> Previous research shows that health professionals' beliefs about the father's labouring role and the way they treat men can influence the man's assessment of his own needs, the information and support he receives, how involved he feels in the process, and how comfortable he is giving support to his partner.[23]

It then appears that it may be within the mother's control to invite the father into involvement, and that her views about what makes a man 'man enough' may then have an influence on the father's level of involvement. The mother's endorsement of the father's masculinity may act to indemnify the father against his self-consciousness about trespassing into the 'milky world'.

As inferred earlier in the section dealing with the value to children of involved fathers, which examined the effect that they have on their children's attitudes to gender stereotypes, the mother may be more likely to offer this indemnity if she was brought up in a family with a positively involved father herself. This has been confirmed by separate research. As Burgess puts it:

> a woman's relationship with her own father can be *more* significant than her partner's to his father, in predicting his degree of participation, as can be her attitude to non-traditional roles for men.

The mother's power to influence how involved the father becomes is generally known as 'gatekeeping':

> Mothers are gatekeepers, capable of enhancing or dampening father–infant attachment. . . . If they promote a triangle, this opens the way for the child's future attachment.[24]

The mother's potential to act as gatekeeper again emphasises the significance for health professionals of an acknowledgement of the relationship between the parents (and not just the mother–child or father–child relationship), which was noted in the context of the impact of the father's attitude to breastfeeding and both partners' attitudes to smoking during pregnancy.

What may be required is a change of emphasis from suggestions made to both parents that the father should act in a supporter role (which may encourage mothers to act as restrictive gatekeepers of the father's involvement), to a less interven-tionist facilitation of the formation of such a triangle or parenting partnership by dialogue between the parents.

In practical terms, the couple should be encouraged to discuss their expectations and the father should be given an opportunity to voice his expectations. If health professionals are seen to promote such a dialogue – removing the automatic suggestion that the father should act only as supporter — it is argued that this will have a beneficial effect. To give the father a point of focus and the opportunity to voice his expectations, and the mother a chance to hear them, in a context where the health professional's promotion of such a dialogue affords proper legitimacy to the father's expression of his views as a prospective parent, might itself facilitate the formation of such a triangle.

As Marcy White suggested in an analysis of men's concerns during pregnancy:

> open communication between the husband and wife regarding the father's role should be encouraged during the prenatal period so that the couple is able to reach a mutual understanding regarding their expectations.[25]

In any event, facilitating communication between the partners cannot be regarded as contentious. After all, it is the relationship between the parents that is the context in which the child's development occurs.

What men report about their attitudes and needs

- Fathers have their own motivations for and attitudes to parenthood, as well as being subject to structural forces.
- These will often express themselves by reference to commonly held concepts associated with fatherhood, such as responsibility and the role of supporter.

It is as well to emphasise, as Burgess goes on to point out, that fathers also have their own autonomous motivations that are distinct from the mother's expectations. For example, they can be driven to compensate for bad relationships with their own fathers, as well as often responding to incidental need where health problems give rise to impediments to the mother's parenting.

Responsibility: what men say

- The concept of responsibility is often associated with fatherhood.
- However, its application is so broad that it is subject to specific interpretation by fathers.
- Although responsibility is a concept that fathers subscribe to, its meaning for them is not just interpreted as financial responsibility or the breadwinner role, and includes the interpretation of caring.
- Practitioners may benefit from exploring fathers' individual interpretations of the concept of responsibility, rather than assuming that they wish to adopt the breadwinner role exclusively.

In particular, a major motivating factor for men is found in the concept of 'responsibility'. For example, as the study by Williams found, 'while fathers may articulate the meaning of fatherhood in diverse ways, the concept of "responsibility" is the dominant emerging concept, a potentially important focus for health promotion with fathers.'[26]

This might appear on the face of it to confirm traditional views about fatherhood, seeming perhaps to focus on the father's breadwinning role. However, it is argued above that men have a limited shared vocabulary to draw upon for expressing concepts of parenting to themselves and with which they feel able to discuss concepts of parenting among themselves (*see* p. 25 on enabling a positive masculinity). However, it should not be stereotypically assumed that men as individuals, using a personal rather than a shared vocabulary, are unable to talk about such concepts.

The difference in the shared and individual vocabulary of men's parenting is highlighted in William's identification of the salience of 'responsibility' as a key theme in the responses of the men whom he surveyed. Concepts of parenting associated with men (but not always by men) often coalesce quickly around a very limited range of keywords, including 'responsibility', 'support' and 'rights'. Nonetheless, as Williams points out, the men themselves in his study articulate the meaning of fatherhood in diverse rather than limited ways.

What this suggests is that the range of concepts of parenting associated with men is limited by factors other than what men themselves specifically articulate about fatherhood. Men's reluctance to articulate may sometimes be a factor. A deficit of skilled male listeners – unaware of the often succinct and sometimes codified way in which men often articulate – may be another. This emphasises the importance of health professionals listening to what fathers are saying before jumping to conclusions and placing interpretations on their words that may not adequately reflect their intended meaning.

Closer examination of the meaning of the term 'responsibility' found in the study by Williams reveals, for example, that for the men in the study, the term actually encompasses several concepts (bringing money into the home, providing security or guidance, and providing protection, care, and help with children's learning).[27]

Thus a key word in the debate about fatherhood, namely responsibility, often associated with one aspect of fatherhood, namely breadwinning, can be found to have a multiplicity of meanings beyond that single aspect, yet these (like much fathering) remain largely hidden. Notable in the meanings found on closer examination is the concept of care. What Williams' identification of the theme of responsibility may mean is that the men are expressing the desire to act as a principally engaged parent, enacting their parenting function in a variety of ways, rather than a desire or willingness to act in a secondary or merely supportive capacity.

The supporter role: what men say

- The supporter role is another concept that is broadly applied to men and fatherhood.
- Men subscribe to this role, but it is interpreted in different ways by individual fathers, and includes emotional as well as financial meanings.

- Fathers can express their wish to be involved in their families by reference to the concept of support, but this does not imply that they accept marginalisation as parents.
- The heavy scripting of the supporter role for fathers tends to result in their own information needs not being met.
- Emphasis on men's supporter role acts to undermine the autonomy of men's parenting.

Support is another key concept that is applied to fatherhood, and its meanings and application have been examined above. Although it is acknowledged that this is a role with which men identify, it is suggested that the role is heavily scripted. Closer examination of what men say is again instructive.

'Supporting your family' is a phrase associated with the male breadwinning role, positing for the father a somewhat external situation in relation to his family, but the word 'support' in its present-day application has acquired emotional in addition to purely financial content.

For example, for the young fathers who were interviewed in the Prince's Trust report, *It's Like That: the views and hopes of disadvantaged young people*, one of the clear priorities for good fathering, indeed the first, was providing support for mother and child, 'emotionally and financially'.[28] This expresses a desire for involvement with the family that does not merely include earning an income for the family.

During their partner's pregnancy men provide most support for their partners, and the National Childbirth Trust survey found that they are less likely to share their own concerns with their partners. However, in addition to suggesting that these men may lack the opportunity to discuss their concerns, the survey makes it clear that this is subject to more than the simple interpretation that men adopt the supporter role because this is what they would choose in any case:

> many men suggested that they were less likely to share their own concerns with their partners than vice versa. This may mean that men have less opportunity to discuss their worries and have their information and support needs met. Alternatively, it may indicate that men feel less of a desire to talk about their concerns.[a]

It does not follow from this, of course, that men adopt the supporter role willingly on the grounds that they feel less desire to talk about their concerns. They may feel that sharing their concerns with their partner would undermine the support which they give their partner, by adding to their partner's concerns. Indeed, it is on the grounds that men do actually add to their partner's anxieties in this way by burdening them with their own worries that Michel Odent and others argue that they should be excluded from the delivery room.

It has been found that men feel they provide a vital emotional support for their partners as a 'sturdy oak'[29] with whom the mother can 'talk things through.' And men, as the National Childbirth Trust survey found, have significant concerns about their partner and their baby in the perinatal period. They also have worries about money:

---

[a] NCT Survey, p. iv

Previous research has suggested that many men suffer from increased stress and anxiety during their partner's pregnancy.[30] Research has also shown that men's primary concerns centre around the health and safety of their partner and baby.[25] In line with this, the men in the Access survey [i.e. this NCT survey] said that during pregnancy they worried most about 'something being wrong with the baby/tests and scans.' The possibility of miscarriage was also a concern. ... Half of the men were very worried about these two issues. More than a quarter were very worried about money and benefit problems, supporting their partner enough, and their partner's mood swings.[a]

More than a third of men were very worried about how their partner would cope with pain during labour, the possibility of having a caesarean section, things not going as planned, having a cut or tear, and not knowing when their partner had gone into labour. ... One in ten were worried about being sick or 'put off' during the birth.[b]

In contrast with previous studies,[30] there were some differences in how worried men from different groups were. ... Men under 20 and those from lower socio-economic groups were more concerned about pregnancy issues, whereas first-time fathers were more worried about labour and life with a new baby.[c]

However, the survey also notes that men express the need for 'as much information as possible' in the period before and after the birth – that is, more than they are provided with at present:

Men want more information about many issues to do with pregnancy, birth and the postnatal period. Many men indicated that they wanted to know 'as much as possible' in order to support their pregnant partners and for their own understanding and peace of mind. More than two-fifths of men wanted to find out more about:

- the choices that exist regarding maternity care services
- reasons for and what to expect with assisted deliveries and caesareans
- ways that their pregnant partner could help herself regarding pain relief during the birth
- postnatal depression
- money and benefits
- coping with a lack of sleep
- the baby's crying and sleeping
- coping with the baby and other children
- the effect of the baby on their relationship with their partner.[d]

However, the survey also goes on to suggest that this thirst for information could be an indicator of needs of their own:

It is important to note that just because men say they want more information does not necessarily mean that they need more written material or more facts and figures. Instead, this could be a way of expressing a

---

[a] NCT Survey, p. 37; [b] p. 38; [c] p. 39; [d] p. 34

desire for greater support or reassurance about different topics, or more opportunity to discuss their concerns, have their questions answered, gain reassurance or alleviate their anxieties. This possibility is supported by previous research.[31]

Overall, therefore, men feel that they provide a vital emotional support to their partners, but closer inspection of the supporter role reveals that they have a whole range of concerns of their own. It is also reasonable to conclude, given that many of their anxieties are about the health and safety of their partner, that they lend support to their partner not because they have no concerns of their own, but precisely in order to address some of their own concerns just as they censor the expression of their own anxieties for this reason.

Thus even where men are perceived to subscribe to the supporter role, heavily scripted as it is for men by health professionals, they do so in order to address their autonomous concerns as principally engaged parents, and not as acceptance of secondary status as parents. They also have many concerns of their own. Both observations support their engagement as principally engaged parents, just as with their identification with the concept of responsibility. Men's nominal acceptance of the role of supporter should not therefore be misinterpreted and taken as grounds upon which to treat them as a secondary type of parent with no proper, principally engaged concerns.

The findings of the National Childbirth Trust survey with regard to antenatal classes also 'support previous research which suggests that men want to be acknowledged as one half of the parental duo'.[32] However, perhaps the position for men with regard to the supporter role is best summed up by Nina Smith's analysis of men's needs in these classes:

> Classes were judged to have played a positive and indispensable role for men when they addressed the issues of the man as a labour supporter *and also affirmed him as an involved parent* [my italics]. Regardless of how things worked out in practice, when these issues were ignored, the men felt that classes were a waste of time.[33]

Nor is there any justification for excluding men from the information loop where the focus remains on their supporter role, given that they are the most heavily relied upon support system for women during pregnancy.[34]

Andrea Robertson also argued in *The Practising Midwife* that meeting men's own needs is itself necessary in order for them to provide good support:

> It is unfair to expect them to provide practical help and emotional support if their own needs have not been met, and if they have no training in what to do.[35]

Fathers in the delivery room

- Most fathers attend the birth of their children, and their presence at the birth is broadly accepted by professionals, subject to their supporter role.
- Fathers' approaches to their presence at the birth take a variety of forms and reveal heterogeneity among fathers.

> - Dialogue between the couple beforehand in order to develop joint expectations of the father's approach enhances the experience for both parents.
> - For professionals, facilitating such a dialogue is as important at the time of the birth as at other times, and may establish a pattern of dialogue that enhances mutual understanding between the parents for the future.

As Deborah Ghate, Catherine Shaw and Neal Hazel made clear in an analysis of the use of family centres by fathers,[36] men are not a homogenous group, and just as they articulate the meanings of key concepts of fatherhood in different ways, in the period before and after the birth they have different individual needs and expectations. The focus of these differences is perhaps found in the men's expectations of their attendance at the birth.

Burgess cites the work of Jackson, who identified four categories of expectant father:

> Jackson developed four categories for the fathers he met. In addition to the *refusers* (20 per cent), there were the *spectators* (20 per cent) who were fundamentally supportive but professed themselves unaffected ('We've both seen babies on TV, so it'll be alright I should think') and the *sharers*, who were the great majority (50 per cent), who said things like 'No, I've never been to the hospital or these classes. I wait till Liz comes back and then I want all the news'. The final group were the *identifiers* (10 per cent), who tried to experience the whole thing with their wives.[37]

'Refusers' were identified as follows:

> Brian Jackson interviewed 100 married or cohabiting fathers to be in the early 1980s, and found that one in five were extremely hostile to their partner's pregnancy. Jackson called the unwilling fathers in his sample 'refusers', and it is interesting to note that the one in five refusers mirrors the one in five pregnancies that women have terminated.[38]

Incidentally, Burgess notes the value Jackson suggested of providing information for the father when promoting paternal involvement among these men:

> Counselling and educating fathers at this stage can pay off in other ways, improving the quality of father–child attachment, mother–child involvement and breastfeeding rates. Jackson felt that, with proper antenatal preparation, many of the fathers he interviewed would have moved a category closer to involvement – refusers to spectators, spectators to sharers, and so on.[39]

Marcy White cites the work of Chapman, who identified 'three separate roles assumed by men during labour and birth: coach, teammate and witness.' White goes on to explain the meaning of these definitions for Chapman:

> Men in the role of coach viewed themselves as managers or directors of the labour experience, and their partners wanted them to have an active

and physically involved role. Teammates assisted their partners through labour by following the needs and directions of others. The teammates' partners had a strong desire for the men to be present and willing to assist them by following their directions or cues. Witnesses, on the other hand, were present primarily to observe the birth of their infant and to be a companion to their partner. For a man to feel comfortable in the role of witness, it was important that his partner's major expectation be that he be present for the experience.[40]

Incidentally, White notes Chapman's observation of the importance of the couple communicating about the 'role of the father', which adds weight to the argument made here that health professionals facilitate and acknowledge dialogue between the expectant parents:

> Chapman (1992) also noted that in order for the couple to view the birth experience as a team effort in which they were working together, it was important for the couple to reach a high degree of mutuality and understanding regarding the role of the father.[41]

It is reasonable to conclude that establishing at the outset a pattern of dialogue between expectant parents about the couple's expectations of the father's presence at the birth will assist in establishing a pattern of dialogue about their parenting that will benefit their partnership after the birth as well.

Informing fathers: men's groups?

- In seeking to include fathers in the information loop, practitioners may consider establishing a men's group.
- Prior to the birth, however, men's heterogeneity with regard to their expectations of their presence in the delivery room may inhibit communication in such groups.
- Later, men's lack of a common parenting vocabulary may also inhibit the functioning and value of such groups.
- Men may be suspicious about such groups.
- Practitioners who are unsure about men's needs and how to support them should not necessarily assume that men will want to support each other in such groups.
- Fathers respond to the concept of parenthood, rather than to that of fatherhood, and tend not to view parenting in a gender-distinct way which men's groups might otherwise help to define.
- The emphasis should therefore perhaps be placed on promoting dialogue between the two parents.

Observing parents picking up their children at the school gates, it is striking how often one sees the mothers engaged in conversation with each other whereas the fathers rarely acknowledge each others' presence. The more obviously involved fathers will nonetheless often engage in conversation with the mothers.

It is also noteworthy that the National Childbirth Trust survey found that men were less likely to attend antenatal classes in order to meet other parents than were women.[42]

It was suggested earlier that fathers, and men in general, have no shared vocabulary with which to discuss their parenting among themselves, and no templates on which to base or found such discussions. On an individual level, of course, men are perfectly capable of articulating their feelings, although they may often feel that it is not appropriate for them to do so.

This raises the question of whether setting up a father's group is an effective means of disseminating and sharing information and promoting skilled parenting among fathers.

Ghate identified suspicion of men's groups among non-users, and difficulties in the recruitment of users:

> Most of the men who attended had taken a great deal of persuasion to get involved, and all bemoaned the fact that it was hard to recruit new members ... non-users had ambivalent, if not actually negative, views of the groups. We concluded, therefore, that although men's groups are enabling for some, they may not be a first line of service provision. Providing a men's group alone is unlikely to be a successful way to recruit large numbers of fathers. Rather, men's groups should perhaps be viewed as an 'advanced' activity for established users of centres.[43]

These questions about men's/fathers' groups, which are also considered in detail by Lloyd,[44] are in addition reflected in surveys of men during the antenatal period. Nina Smith found similar ambivalent views among non-users and a feeling that that such groups did not reflect the shared nature of parenting:

> Five interviewees gave a definite 'no' to the idea of men-only sessions, considering it totally contrary to the shared nature of the antenatal class experience, which reflected the shared nature of pregnancy, birth and parenthood. ... It was interesting, however, that even the enthusiasts were uncertain about what type of man would attend such a session. Would he in effect be too 'new'?[45]

The National Childbirth Trust survey also found reluctance about men-only groups and other parents' groups among non-users:

> More than two-thirds said that they definitely would not use local fathers' groups/contacts, weekly parent/baby drop-in groups and information for fathers on the Internet.[a]

However, it also found a greater appeal of such groups among the unemployed:

> Approximately one in ten men said they would definitely use local weekend drop-in groups for parents and babies and a national telephone

---

[a] NCT Survey, p. v

helpline for fathers. Up to one in twenty men said they would definitely use weekday drop-in groups or local fathers' groups/contacts. These services were more appealing to fathers who were not employed.[a]

Yet perhaps the principal weakness of fathers' groups in the antenatal context is a sense that to attend such a group gives a definite, unwanted sense of the father being relegated to the parenting 'B' team. This supports the argument made above with regard to men's responses to the concept of the 'supporter role' and that of 'responsibility' – that they fundamentally want to be acknowledged as principally engaged parents, or one half of what the National Childbirth Trust survey called the 'parental duo'. As Nina Smith observed:

> The desire to show commitment was symptomatic of the fact that all interviewees considered the shared nature of contemporary parenthood indisputable. They did not all approve, but there was a general acceptance that traditional gender roles have broken down, and going to antenatal classes together was a manifestation of this, a symbol of the partnership of parenthood.[46]

For health professionals, as with messages such as those which promote breastfeeding, this perhaps again emphasises the need to acknowledge the relationship between the parents themselves, and not to box parents into separate gender groups with unrelated needs. Smith observed that:

> Ideas about shared parenthood meant that learning about parenting together with partners was expected, with gender needs merging. Fatherhood itself was seen as a low priority – *parenthood* was the key concept.[47]

Again the emphasis should perhaps be on facilitating dialogue between the parents about the father's involvement, as was argued above, rather than on separate fathers' groups. As Nina Smith further observes:

> Experience of classes endorsed their views, giving men an opportunity to show commitment and to share more fully with partners. Those disappointed in other areas still considered these valid reasons for attending a course. The key factor was doing this *together*. The chance to set aside formal time in the midst of a busy life to think about the coming baby together was valued, and could be missed when the course ended.[48]

However, all of this is not to say that fathers' groups are never appropriate as a means of supporting fathers. Established groups across the country, although thin on the ground, have demonstrated their value to many fathers experiencing difficulty or otherwise needing support. The experienced and dedicated practitioners who lead such groups are skilled at building trust between group members and using this trust as a therapeutic and learning tool. Members of such groups often report a valued experience where discussing barriers and difficulties that they experience, or problematic behaviour, can be addressed in a positive way.

---

[a] NCT Survey, p. 92

Informing fathers: information content

> - The information needs of expectant mothers and fathers are broadly similar.
> - Existing information designed for mothers can therefore be efficiently tailored and reproduced for fathers, but may benefit from an awareness of masculine perspectives.
> - Providing men with information would relieve mothers of the current burden that falls on them of being the fathers' main source of information.

The National Childbirth Trust survey provides specific advice about the information that men ask for during the perinatal period. Some of the findings are quoted above, and the survey is invaluable for identifying much more of the information that men say they need.

However, it is significant that the survey does not argue for the development of a whole new expertise in information content. On the contrary, in support of Smith's observation about gender needs merging, what it argues for is the need to convey existing knowledge to men, suggesting that men and women want to know about the same things:

> The findings suggest that although there are differences, men and women have similar information needs during pregnancy. There are significant gaps between the information that men want when their partner is pregnant and what they are able to find out. Health professionals should specifically address men's information needs and aim to provide opportunities for men to discuss their questions and concerns.[a]

Thus differences appear to lie not so much in information content as in information delivery method. The merits of fathers' groups as such a method were considered above.

It should be remembered, of course, that asking for information may also be a discreet way of asking for support. However, the above analysis of fathers' groups suggests that men do not have a shared vocabulary or set of conversational templates about parenting on which they could found such mutual support, even supposing that they were predisposed to seek and offer such support among themselves. This supposition is itself open to considerable doubt.

Men also often have difficulty in attending antenatal appointments, either because the latter are scheduled during working hours and they are unable to take time off work, or because they are not made to feel welcome.

It is for these reasons (and others) that men mainly obtain information about pregnancy, birth and parenting from their partner. However, if men are being asked to support women during this period, it does not seem logical to put the burden of informing the father on the mother (except where it is judged that this is a means of allowing the mother to involve the father to the extent that she wishes, as in the view identified by Lavender that it is for the mother and the midwife to determine the role of the father).

---

[a] NCT Survey, p. 35

Thus the question arises as to what is the best means of providing men with the information that they seek in order to be engaged parents, and thereby acknowledging and encouraging them as such. This also includes (but does not consist solely of) answering and allaying their concerns about the health of their baby and partner, which will assist them in providing support to their partners.

If men's groups and antenatal appointments do not always provide the best opportunities, alternative methods of reaching the father with information need to be considered. As the National Childbirth Trust survey notes:

> The take-up of antenatal information among fathers remains low, suggesting a need for a strategic rethink. Fathers should be invited, welcomed and involved when information about birth and babycare is being offered to new parents.[a]

It is an interesting point that being invited, welcomed and involved appears to be as important as the information itself, particularly if men's and women's information needs are largely the same.

Although it is necessary to bear in mind the similarity of men's and women's information needs, it may nonetheless also be important to acknowledge a male perspective in information that is given to the father. This point is addressed in the final section of this chapter.

Informing fathers: father-friendly environments

- Service environments, particularly hospitals, convey their own message to fathers about the value that is attributed to their parenthood.
- An absence of images of fatherhood and an unwelcoming approach by staff can convey as negative a message as the exclusion of the father from the information loop and an excessive emphasis on his supporter role.

The findings of the National Childbirth Trust survey showed that the hospital setting is a key environment for the father. This is where he is most likely to have met one of the midwives before the birth and where he will also be likely to have met a hospital doctor. Fathers are more likely to encounter these professionals in a hospital than in a local community facility.

> The men were most likely to have visited doctors and midwives at hospitals. ... Two-thirds had visited a midwife at the hospital and three-fifths had visited hospital doctors.[b]

The survey suggests the following reasons for fathers' higher level of attendance at hospitals rather than community clinics prior to the birth:

> This may mean that rather than participating in routine visits to midwives and doctors in community settings, men are more likely to attend appointments if there are potential problems with the pregnancy or if

[a] NCT Survey, p. iv; [b] p. 8

issues such as induction are being discussed. It may be considered more acceptable to get time off work in these circumstances. Alternatively, it may mean that hospital appointment times fit more easily into men's schedules or that they welcome the chance to visit the hospital where their baby will be born.[a]

Although the father is very likely to attend for a hospital appointment prior to the birth, there is often little or nothing there to welcome him as an expectant parent. In the waiting-room there will be a range of notices and posters directed at mothers, but very few (if any) featuring an image of a father or addressed to the father as one of the child's parents.

After the waiting-room, there might be some difficulty in finding a chair for the father in the appointment room where the parents discuss the oncoming birth with the midwife or doctor. If there is a chair in the room for the father, it may be anywhere, but the expectant mother is directed to take the chair next to the midwife's or doctor's desk.

What images of fathers involved with their children (displayed in the hospital antenatal settings) achieve, as much as do welcoming and informative approaches of professionals, is to give a message to the father that his parenting is perceived by others to be of value. Equally, the absence of such images and signals imparts its own message – that his parenting is not valued – which can damage relationships between parents and undermine the father's involvement and engagement with his family and children at a crucial developmental stage.

Informing fathers: through direct communication with them

- Giving information to the father through a variety of media has value in itself in acknowledging the father's parenthood.
- Awareness of a masculine perspective in information materials for fathers can be valuable.
- However, caution must be exercised with a view to avoiding stereotypical approaches such as an excessive use of metaphors involving sports or cars, but bearing in mind that such metaphors may be of value in establishing 'common ground' at the outset.
- Generic materials produced for mothers and fathers can fail to appeal to fathers if feminine fonts and colours are used. Parenting materials produced in such a way are rapidly interpreted as being designed exclusively for mothers.
- In such materials, as elsewhere, use of the words 'parent', 'parenting' and 'parenthood' have lost much of their meaning of including mothers and fathers, and are becoming interpreted as excluding fathers.
- Where practitioners encounter few fathers and uptake of printed materials for them is low, outreach projects that take the materials or project information to the fathers outside service environments may be of benefit.

[a] NCT Survey, p. 8

- Relying exclusively on mothers to distribute materials to fathers carries the message to fathers that they are not invited to participate in a dialogue themselves.
- Taking the opportunity to give fathers an information pack at the time of the birth capitalises on their presence and receptiveness.

As in the settings mentioned above, it is suggested that information which is designed to appeal to fathers by including visual images of the latter, and which is expressly worded to include fathers as well as mothers, conveys a direct message to them that their parenting is valued and acknowledged. Equally, the absence of such information conveys the opposite message.

However, apart from his being directly addressed in visual materials, no more direct message can be conveyed of the acknowledgement of a father as a parent than by his being physically handed information that affirms him as such. Yet current methods of distribution of the very few materials (including *The Bounty Guide to Fatherhood*) that are addressed directly to the father are themselves indirect in that they rely on the mother to pass the materials on to him.

This in itself could be said to convey a message to both parents about the father's status. Why was he not given the materials himself? Again the distribution of materials to the father via the mother — like the suggestion by health professionals that the role of the father is that of supporter to the mother, rather than of a prospective new parent himself — emphasises the primacy of the mother's parenting. It also burdens the mother with the task of informing the father, and may suggest to the father that he is not invited into a dialogue himself, whether or not that is something he wants.

It should be noted here that distribution methods can impact contextually on the meaning of the content of the information that is being distributed. The previous paragraph explains how this can happen. However, by way of further example, a pamphlet about cot death which may already be produced in feminine fonts and colours, included in an information pack that is handed exclusively to mothers on discharge, may be perceived as being the proper concern of mothers by a father who is looking through that information, by virtue of the fact that the pack is handed to and produced for the mother.

In terms of content as distinct from distribution, Smith's finding that it is often the concept of *parenthood* that appeals to men, rather than *fatherhood per se*, is also worth bearing in mind when producing information for fathers. Equally worth noting are her findings, and those of the National Childbirth Trust survey, that the information needs of men and women are substantially the same.

However, this should be set against Ghate's findings that men need acknowledgement of issues pertaining to their masculinity. The National Childbirth Trust survey also finds that men 'also wanted material that explored their concerns from a male perspective.'[a]

The distribution of authentically generic materials which are made available and distributed directly to men and women would therefore appear to be part of a solution. However, if materials are distributed to men they may also benefit from

[a] NCT Survey, p. 33

being aware of a male perspective. The material for new fathers may therefore need to contain two different elements – first, the theme of parenthood rather than fatherhood, but secondly, on an individual level, an acknowledgment of the implications of being male for fathers.

However, attention must again be paid to Ghate's parallel finding that men do not represent a homogenous group. Men vary widely as individuals and also, as shown above (*see* p. 68), they do not necessarily like football. Therefore giving materials a masculine tone need not always mean heavily theming them around sport in general or football in particular. Nonetheless, although it was argued in Chapter 2 that men differ widely as individuals from the 'kitemark' of masculine identity, there are some common templates of masculine conversations which men can share as a convenient tool for establishing common ground. The occasional use of sporting, motoring or IT metaphors may to this extent be appropriate.

Any number of 'guides for new parents' or 'handbooks of parenthood' that are available in bookshops or on 'parenting' websites currently purport to attempt the generic approach. However, they frequently suffer from a lack of authenticity. Often they are simply cosmetic reissues of older publications which were aimed at new motherhood, with a 'dad's section' having been subsequently added at the instigation of the publisher (who prefers not to commission a whole new book).

The problem that arises in these books is that motherhood elides into parenthood, but the father remains as 'dad'. By inference, he therefore fails to qualify for the status of a proper parent. This patronising approach, confining the father to the 'B team' of parenthood, directly contradicts fathers' wishes to be regarded as an integral part of the parenting duo.

The National Childbirth Trust survey found that, after their partners, men mainly used books, magazines, television and radio programmes, leaflets, friends and antenatal classes as sources of information. One in five (i.e. substantially fewer) obtained information from videos. The level of use of the Internet was found to be very low, but might now be growing. Succinct printed answers to frequently asked questions, with a practical emphasis, particularly by authors viewed as experts, were also highly valued.

However, it must be noted that many such information sources fail to serve men's needs, attendant visual cues revealing that the content actually contains very little that includes the father. On websites in particular this can often be due as much to the colours and design of the product advertisements that pop up on the front page as to the colours and graphic design of the website itself. Conversely, fathers can equally be led away from material that is substantively inclusive of them by the colours and graphic design (or indeed the title) of publications and the advertisements that they feature.

For those few projects that are currently working with fathers, the question is always how to reach them. Services that are considering working with fathers are also now beginning to ask the same question. For example, in Australia a men's health project goes to stock car races and offers 'health MOTs' to men.[49] In a report in which Yvette Cooper, Junior Health Minister, acknowledged that the greatest health inequality in the UK in 2000 was that between men and women – and it was the *men* who were underprovided for – it was shown that services may have to be taken out to men, rather than waiting for them to talk to a GP or nurse. This has led to men's health clinics being held in pubs and betting shops in the West Midlands.[50]

Inventive and imaginative as these approaches are, and complex as the issues are for some services for men, if hospitals and family support services working in collaboration with them see the virtues of including new fathers in the process of their work, the least difficulty they will encounter is in bringing these fathers in through the doors. Nine out of ten fathers attend the birth of their children and many attend antenatal appointments before the birth. This amounts to an enormous opportunity to reach men and to start them on a path of inclusion and involvement with their families – an opportunity which must be seized.

It is argued that the distribution of information directly to fathers is as important as style and content in reaching fathers. In attempts that have been made to date, a major hurdle has been men's reluctance or inability to come to antenatal appointments (for reasons examined elsewhere above, where of course it is noted that if their first experience is of a father-friendly environment which they feel invited to enter, the reluctance factor will be reduced). However, it has been found that men will prioritise coming to scans prior to the birth.

The essential argument of this book is that the best opportunity for accessing fathers (or 'reaching' them, in the jargon) is presented by the very significant numbers of fathers who attend the birth. This opportunity arises both in the practical sense that their physical presence allows information to be conveyed to them directly, and also in the sense that their receptiveness and openness at this time make it most likely that they will benefit from the information that they are given. An opportunity is also presented by the increased likelihood of men attending scans prior to the birth.

However, to concentrate on the primal moment of the birth, if fathers cannot take their partners and babies home with them on the first evening (assuming that the hospital has no overnight facilities for fathers), the opportunity can be taken to offer them useful and affirming information to take home with them that recognises and capitalises on the marvel of the moment. In Australia, this approach has been taken by the Men in Families project at Coffs Harbour, where as part of a family support services programme all new fathers are given a simple information pack which includes the contact details of project support workers whom they can contact. Details of the project are given in Appendix 1.

An opportunity might arise at this point, when physically handing the father such an information pack, to iron out any anxieties that he might report that arose during the delivery. Of course, careful consideration must be given to how this might be handled and whether, for example, it should be done by a midwife or other professional who attended the birth, or by someone else who might be regarded as a more neutral figure.

Another point that should be made about the importance of the birth arises from the impact that it can have on the father afterwards. The argument made here is that this represents a case for 'joined-up' care and support for fathers between the hospital, visiting midwives and health visitors and family support projects. One example is found in the Coffs Harbour project, where the local health authority distributes the project's 'Glory Bag' to new fathers.

In this respect it is suggested that family support projects that are working to promote men's positive involvement with their families and maternity services can collaborate with and learn from each other. Maternity services, ironically, have the men coming through their doors to attend the birth. The projects have experience of men's issues and how to support them. Maternity services also have much to contribute to the substance of informing family support with awareness of mothers' issues. The birth must be acknowledged as a key moment for families and a key forum for collaboration by health professionals and agencies supporting families.

References and notes

1   When the author attended one antenatal appointment prior to the birth of his second child he asked whether fathers were allowed to stay overnight, and was told that this was not possible. When he asked why, intending to explore the midwife's and the hospital's attitudes and policy about fathers, he was told that, apart from privacy issues, they were felt to be a 'security risk'. Incidents of theft and drunkenness were alluded to, but the author was discouraged from asking about these incidents. He did not press the issue as he did not want to prejudice the relationship between the midwife and his pregnant partner.

2   Williams R (1999) 'Going the Distance': fathers, health and health visiting. University of Reading, Reading, in association with the Queen's Nursing Institute, London, p. 22.

3   Daniel B and Taylor J (2001) Engaging with Fathers: practice issues for health and social care. Jessica Kingsley Publishers, London, p. 21.

4   Office for Standards in Education (2002) Sex and Relationships. HMI 433. A Report from the Office of Her Majesty's Chief Inspector of Schools; www.ofsted.gov.uk

5   Brunt S (2001) Fathers in Child Protection: a brief look at the current situation. National Society for the Prevention of Cruelty to Children, London.

6   Daniel B and Taylor J, op. cit., p. 21, cite the work of Gilligan R (1998) Men in Foster Care: a case of neglect?, finding that 'Agencies can become "locked into" a conscious or unconscious "risk view" of all fathers.'

7   Daniel B and Taylor J, op. cit., p. 26.

8   Daniel B and Taylor J, op. cit., p. 24.

9   Daniel B and Taylor J, op. cit., p. 26.

10   Lloyd T (2001) What Works with Fathers? Working With Men, London, p. 13.

11   Williams R, op. cit., p. 23.

12   In 1964, the author's father-in-law was only allowed to do this when given a letter of recommended authorisation by his GP, to be given to the hospital.

13   Williams R, op. cit., p. 24, citing Connell R (1995) Masculinities. Polity Press, Cambridge.

14   Ghate D, Shaw C and Hazel N (2000) Fathers and Family Centres. Joseph Rowntree Foundation, York.

15   Lloyd T, op. cit., p. 10.

16   Office for National Statistics (2001) Social Focus on Men. Office for National Statistics, London.

17   FatherFacts, Volume 1, Issue 1 (2001) Fathers Direct, Newpin Fathers Support Centre, NFPI and Working With Men, London, pp. 6 and 7.

18   FatherFacts, op. cit., p. 6.

19   FatherFacts, op. cit., p. 11 (footnote 28).

20   Davidson N and Lloyd T (2001) Boys' and Young Men's Health: practice examples. Stage 1 interim report. Working With Men, for the Health Development Agency, London.

21 Burgess A (1998) *Fatherhood Reclaimed*. Vermillion, London, p. 110.
22 Watson WJ, Watson L, Wetzel W *et al.* (1995) Transition to parenthood. What about fathers? *Can Fam Physician*. **41**: 807–12.
23 NCT Survey, op. cit., p. 55, citing, inter alia, Lester A and Moorston S (1997) Do men need midwives? Facilitating a greater involvement in parenting. *Br J Midwifery*. **5**: 678–86.
24 Burgess A, op. cit., p. 133, citing Brazelton TB and Cramer BG (1991) *The Earliest Relationship*. Karnac, London. 'Gatekeeping' by mothers has also been identified in the National Child Development Study. *See* Joseph Rowntree Foundation (2000) *A Man's Place in the Home: fathers and families in the UK*. Joseph Rowntree Foundation, York, p. 6.
25 White MB (1998) Men's concerns during pregnancy. Part 1. Re-evaluating the role of the expectant father. *Int J Childbirth Educ*. **13**: 14–17.
26 Williams R, op. cit., p. 22.
27 Williams R, op. cit., p. 8.
28 The Prince's Trust (2001) *It's Like That: the views and hopes of disadvantaged young people*. The Prince's Trust, London, p. 28.
29 Lewis C (1986) *Becoming a Father*. Open University Press, Milton Keynes.
30 Thomas SG and Upton D (2000) Expectant fathers' attitudes towards pregnancy. *Br J Midwifery*. **8**: 218–21.
31 NCT Survey, op. cit., p. 34, citing Curtis L (1989) *The First Year of Life: promoting the health of babies in the community*. Maternity Alliance, London.
32 NCT Survey, p. 18.
33 Smith N (1999) Men in antenatal classes: teaching the whole birth thing. *Pract Midwife*. **2**: 23–6.
34 Singh D and Newburn M (eds) (2000) *Access to Maternity Information and Support. The needs and experiences of women before and after birth*. National Childbirth Trust, London.
35 Robertson A (1999) Get the fathers involved! The needs of men in pregnancy classes. *Pract Midwife*. **2**: 21–2.
36 Ghate D, Shaw C and Hazel N (2000) *Fathers and Family Centres*. Joseph Rowntree Foundation, York.
37 Burgess A, op. cit., p. 111, citing Jackson B (1984) *Fatherhood*. Allen and Unwin, London.
38 Burgess A, op. cit., p. 108.
39 Burgess A, op. cit., p. 113.
40 White MB, op. cit., p. 15, citing Chapman L (1992) Expectant fathers' roles during labour and birth. *J Obstet Gynecol Neonatal Nurs*. **21**: 114–20.
41 White MB, op. cit., p. 15.
42 'The most common reason men gave for attending antenatal classes involved getting information, preparing for the birth and to prepare for being a parent.... These were the same reasons given in the Access Project survey of pregnant women. However, men were less likely to say that they were attending classes to meet other parents-to-be. Around two in five men said that they attended antenatal classes to meet others, compared to two-thirds of pregnant women' (NCT Survey, op. cit., p. 16). It should be noted that the question related to meeting other parents and not just fathers. Had it done so, it is suggested the margin of difference would be even wider.
43 Ghate D, Shaw C and Hazel N, op. cit., p. 48.

44 Lloyd T, op. cit., pp. 16–19.
45 Smith N (1999) Antenatal classes and the transition to fatherhood: a study of some fathers' views. *MIDIRS Midwifery Digest.* **9**: 463–8.
46 Smith N, op. cit., p. 463.
47 Smith N, op. cit., p. 465.
48 Smith N, op. cit., p. 463.
49 Squires N (2001) Australian MoT checks oil, plugs and exhaust – of men. *Electronic Telegraph.* **18 March**.
50 Internet site to make better men; *BBC News Online (Health)*, 14 November 2000.

CHAPTER 5

Hospital midwife checklist

Below is a list of suggested father-friendly practice points for the hospital or other health professional service departments.

- Is a chair provided for partners in antenatal appointment and scan rooms?
- Simple greetings and eye contact also convey to partners a sense of welcome and involvement with the expected child. Scan technicians have a role to play here, too.
- Are there images of fathers as well as of mothers visible in the service environment and in the pamphlets, notices and literature that are on display?
- Have any surveys been conducted on fathers' needs? Surveys are more frequently undertaken into mothers' needs, and fathers' needs can be overlooked. Assessing these needs can be a valuable part of a more father-friendly approach, but it should be recognised that the sense fathers have of being welcomed (or discouraged) by the service environment and staff may influence their expectations. Men may also be guarded when completing written surveys, and for this reason surveys on their own may not be a reliable measure for assessing fathers' needs.
- Attitudes towards fathers are important. Are there any attitudes that inhibit a more inclusive approach towards fathers? Consider resolving these with encouragement and promotion of the partner's role, particularly in recognition of the fact that inclusion and support during the antenatal period and the time around the birth are significant for the foundation of the family as a mutually supportive unit.
- Be aware of factors that inhibit fathers' visible involvement. Fathers often prefer to engage in parenting gestures and displays of affection towards their children in private because of a reluctance to engage in ostensibly 'feminine' behaviours, and increasingly because of apprehension about accusations of child abuse. Therefore an apparently aloof attitude displayed by a father should not necessarily be construed as a sign of lack of involvement as a parent.

    Furthermore, if a father's experience of attending antenatal appointments and other visits to the service environment is one of being marginalised and excluded, he will tend to withdraw. Therefore the reasons for such withdrawal need to be assessed before assuming that the father is not interested and excluding him on these grounds.
- Explain the absence of the father's name on the baby's nametag and cot card. The name of the mother, but not that of the father, are included on the newborn's nametag, often to allow quick identification of the child and mother inpatient pair in a fire emergency. However, if this is not explained to the father, the absence of his name on the baby's nametag can create a sense of exclusion.

Similarly, the father's name may not be included on cot cards and birthweight records that are given to new parents. If the father's name is not included explaining the reasons for this can mitigate the sense of exclusion.

- When giving feeding advice and other information to new parents on discharge, aim to hand the fathers advice that is accessible to them as well. Graphic design details such as fonts, images and colour schemes can give implicit visual cues that parenting advice materials are intended to be read by one gender or the other. Men in particular value succinct and expert advice, but in health matters these are valued by all parents. A valuable guide is to be found in *Reaching Parents: Producing and Delivering Parent Information Resources*, published by the National Family and Parenting Institute.

- Anticipate the delivery and early parenting in 'hands-off' discussion with both parents – encouraging a joint dialogue between the parents. Also consider offering fathers the opportunity to cut the umbilical cord, and offer both parents skin-to-skin contact with the newborn. Cutting the cord in particular can come as something of a surprise if it has not been discussed before. Consider offering these options as a route to asking both the father and the mother to be about their joint expectations of how they want to approach the birth (mothers may also want to think about the value of skin-to-skin contact). Fathers may sometimes prefer to avoid seeing too much blood, placenta, etc., and may prefer to stay near their partner's head.

- Consider exercising caution in prescribing the supporter role for the father in such discussions, as this may imply that he has a secondary role as a parent after the birth. This may undermine his involvement (and in effect the support that he gives the mother). Encouraging a dialogue between the parents about their expectations of the birth may help to establish a dialogue about their parenting later. Breastfeeding may be a useful topic to anticipate here, as the nature of the couple's joint expectations and the father sensing that he has a stake in its benefits for his child may increase the likelihood of successful breastfeeding.

  The couple's relationship and an aware and informed father are also important in cases where the mother suffers from postnatal depression.[1]

- Include fathers in teaching about caring (e.g. bathing babies in the evenings so that fathers can attend).[2] Similarly, antenatal classes and other appointments could be scheduled to coincide with a time when the father is able to attend.

- Consider a partnership with a local family support project working with fathers to distribute information and provide support to the father after the birth.

References

1   Aiken C and George M (2000) *Surviving Postnatal Depression*. Jessica Kingsley Publishers, London.
2   Fathers Direct (2002) *FatherFacts. Volume 1. Issue 2. How to build new dads*. Fathers Direct, London.

CHAPTER 6

Health visitor and visiting midwife checklist

Below is a list of suggested father-friendly practice points for health professionals visiting the home environment.

- Consider making telephone appointments that introduce the service as the health visitor or midwife 'for the new baby' rather than expressing it as 'the health visitor for the new mum'.
- Suggest that appointments be made when the father can be present.
- Make it clear from eye contact and greetings that the intention is for the father, too, to have an opportunity to ask questions.
- Attitudes towards fathers are important. Are there any attitudes that inhibit a more inclusive approach to fathers? Consider resolving these with encouragement and promotion of the partner's role, particularly in recognition of the fact that inclusion and support during the antenatal period and the time around the birth are significant for the foundation of the family as a mutually supportive unit.
- Collect information about the father as well. Consider starting the conversation by asking him whether he was present at the birth and, if so, why he wanted to attend. His answer might say something about his general expectations of fatherhood or link into issues that he might want to raise.
- At present, parents' copies of child health and immunisation records contain the undertaking that 'your details as the natural mother will only be disclosed to your family doctor and health visitor'. Clearly this is undermining for fathers who are taking their children to be immunised, to the GP or to well baby clinics. Look at all literature from the perspective of accessibility in this way.
- Do not assume a lack of knowledge or competence from the father. It may be that he has been closely involved in events leading up to the birth and has a high level of knowledge. Even if this is not the case, giving the father the impression that he is expected to be ill informed and lacking in competence conveys a negative message about what is expected of him.
- Do not thank the father for involved actions that he undertakes, such as changing a nappy, because this implies that he is doing something which is not his job.
- Seek information about local family support projects that are supportive of fathers for referrals where required.
- Anticipate early parenting in 'hands-off' discussion with both parents, encouraging a joint parenting dialogue between the couple. Consider exercising caution in prescribing the supporter role for the father in such discussions, as this may imply that he has a secondary role as a parent after the birth. This may undermine his involvement (and in effect the support that he gives the mother).

Encouraging a dialogue between the parents about their expectations of early parenthood may help to establish a dialogue about their parenting. Breastfeeding may be a useful topic to address here, as the nature of the couple's joint expectations and the father sensing that he has a stake in its benefits for his child may increase the likelihood of successful breastfeeding.

The couple's relationship and an aware and informed father are also important in cases where the mother suffers from postnatal depression.[1]

- Be aware of factors that inhibit fathers' visible involvement. Fathers often prefer to engage in parenting gestures and displays of affection towards their children in private or when they are not being observed, because of a reluctance to engage in ostensibly 'feminine' behaviours and increasingly because of apprehension about accusations of child abuse. Therefore an apparently aloof attitude displayed by a father should not necessarily be construed as a sign of lack of involvement as a parent.

Reference

1   Aiken C and George M (2000) *Surviving Postnatal Depression.* Jessica Kingsley Publishers, London.

CHAPTER 7

Family support services checklist

Below is a list of suggested father-friendly practice points for family support services working with families around the time of the birth.

- Treat the birth as a key moment of potential to support the participation of the father in the family from the outset.
- Remember that although working with fathers often requires appreciation of issues relating to masculinity, fathers can nonetheless identify themselves as parents, rather than as fathers as a distinct class of parent.
- Written materials and information distributed around the time of the birth must negotiate between these two requirements – acknowledging the father's masculinity but not stereotyping him as a football and car fanatic.
- The father, just like the mother, becomes a new parent in the context of their relationship. Some appreciation of the dynamics and context of that relationship may assist the delivery of appropriate support to the father that will be constructive in the context of that relationship.
- Fathers' groups may not always be the best medium for providing support at this stage. New fathers in particular may well not share a common parenting vocabulary that is suitable for the functioning of such a group. However, these groups can be of great therapeutic value for some fathers.
- Consider exploring with the father why he attended or did not attend the birth. This may link into his expectations of parenthood.
- Men may borrow key terms and phrases such as 'supporter' and 'responsibility', but often they have their own interpretation of what terms such as these mean. It may be necessary to exercise caution by not assuming that the father means what the worker understands the term to mean, and to be certain of what the father himself means by the use of such terms.
- Ultimately, conveying a sense of valuing fathers and what they can bring to their families may be vital – without necessarily attempting to fundamentally re-engineer or change them. Such an approach can key into the father's positive potential and give him the confidence to be the parent he wants to be.

CHAPTER 8

Books on fatherhood

There are currently few books that focus on the enormous potential value of accessing men at a time when they are known to be particularly receptive, namely before and after the birth, within the context of providing solutions in the debate about problematic aspects of masculinity and fatherhood. This book is therefore intended to be distinct in that it suggests a preventative approach by starting off fathers' engagement with their families on the solution track, and offering specific guidance to this end, rather than taking a problem-focused or remedial approach when things go wrong later.

For the general reader there are currently many books written by fathers, or by sons about their fathers, or by other authors on the theme of fatherhood. Authors include Patrick Augustus, Jonathan Myerson, Fay Weldon, Matthew Carr, Blake Morrison, Art Spiegelman, John O'Farrell, Mark Barrowcliffe, Tony Parsons, Jonathan Self, Phil Hogan, Nick Hornby, Colin Shindler, John Lewis Stempel, Peter Howarth, Charles Jennings, Simon Carr and Alan Titchmarsh.

Being aimed at the general reader, rather than at practitioners, managers and policy makers, these books tend to speak of individual experiences and biographies rather than assessing the needs of new and expectant fathers. Sometimes becoming a father has caused the authors to reflect on their own relationships with their fathers, often regretting how disengaged fathers of that generation were. However, these books, some of which might be described as 'dadlit' as well as others that take a more factual and (auto)biographical approach, all tend to attest to a growing identification with parenthood by men. This itself supports the argument that the needs of individual fathers (but in practice not just middle-class consumers of literature) should be recognised and met by health and family services.

There are also family policy and research publications that have appeared in the UK within the last decade (e.g. from the Institute of Public Policy Research, the Policy Research Bureau, the Home Office Family Policy Unit, the Family Policy Studies Centre and the Joseph Rowntree Foundation), some of which draw on policy developments and family studies in the USA, such as the Families and Work Institute, that argue for a recognition of the changing role of fathers within families and for fathers to be valued for more than their pay packets. Conversely, it is recognised that attributing value to fathers' active parenting enables women to play a fuller role in the labour market. This book draws these streams of policy thought into a practical application that facilitates and encourages fathers' active parenting within the contexts of health professionals' and family support workers' practice.

There is another relevant but distinct class of books which could be described as 'parenting' books, that aim to assist and inform individual fathers. These include David Cohen's recent book on fatherhood as well as publications by Fathers Direct, the Maternity Alliance, the National Childbirth Trust, Kevin Osborn and

Rob Parsons. This class of book again attests to fathers' growing participation and interest in active parenting.

There are several publications, in two instances linked with practitioner training courses (*Strengthening Families* and National Center for Strategic Non-profit Planning and Community Leadership (NPCL) sourced training for working effectively with fathers – both US programmes brought in by UK charities), aimed at practitioners in family support services. Both of these programmes aim to train facilitators for parenting or peer support groups and to develop group work.

For professionals and academics who are involved with families and child development, the touchstone book on fatherhood is *The Role of the Father in Child Development* by Michael Lamb, but possibly of equal importance is *How Fathers Care for the Next Generation: a Four-Decade Study* by J Snarey (published by Harvard University Press). This is perhaps of just as much relevance to policy makers in grounding the social benefits of involved fatherhood. A powerful book published in the UK that appeals to fathers, policymakers and practitioners alike is *Fatherhood Reclaimed* by Adrienne Burgess. Ross Parke's books, *Fatherhood* and *Throwaway Dads*, are also well aimed at engaging these audiences, and they translate well from the US to the UK context.

However, the following recent publications which are more narrowly related to the specific subject of this book are highlighted below as being potentially of particular interest.

Singh D and Newburn M (2000) *Becoming a Father*. National Childbirth Trust in association with Fathers Direct, London.

This book contains a great deal of evidence-based research on the expressed information needs of fathers in various settings (in encounters with doctors and midwives in hospitals and community clinics) before and after the birth, and has also served as a valuable source of information for the present book. Its policy recommendations for changes to maternity services to be more inclusive of fathers are also very constructive.

Williams R (1999) *Going the Distance: fathers, health and health visiting*. University of Reading, Reading, in association with the Queen's Nursing Institute, London.

This booklet considers local health visiting practices in the Small Heath area of Birmingham. It argues that services should be expanded so as to be more inclusive of fathers, and it looks at individual fathers' views about parenthood. It also suggests that mother/child-centred service models can reinforce women's caring responsibilities within the home. As such it has served as a source for the present book.

Ryan M (2000) *Working with Fathers*. Radcliffe Medical Press, Oxford.

This book describes the impact of fathers on children's development in problem families, and explores the complex aspects of a father's role, including the legal status of different family situations.

With an emphasis on child protection issues, but with some descriptions of other services available for fathers seeking help, this book mainly addresses the position where there is an existing problem in an individual family.

Lloyd T (2001) *What Works with Fathers?* Working With Men, London.

This book was funded by the Family Policy Unit of the Home Office. Trefor Lloyd from Working With Men is one of the most experienced practitioners in the field.

Working With Men is a not-for-profit organisation that supports the development of work with men through resources, other publications, training and project consultancy.

This book analyses the lessons learned from ten father support projects, and contains a literature review of practice issues. There is some emphasis on group-work projects, and the birth is identified as a key opportunity for accessing men.

Davidson N and Lloyd T (2001) *Boys' and Young Men's Health. Practice examples. Stage 1 interim report.* Working With Men for the Health Development Agency, London.

Available to download free online, www.hda-online.org.uk/yphn, this is a review of several projects, only some of which are addressing the needs of young fathers. The review mainly consists of returns completed by these projects about their goals and working methods. One of several headings of the returns deals with the projects' working assumptions about men, which provide helpful illustrations about the challenges that are facing young fathers. For example, two of the themes that are identified are men's exclusion from traditional health service models *ab initio* or by process, and the importance of issues pertaining to masculinity.

Daniel B and Taylor J (2001) *Engaging with Fathers: Practice Issues for Health and Social Care.* Jessica Kingsley Publishers, London.

This book examines the marginalisation of fathers in child protection practice and the reasons for such prejudice. It offers practice and policy suggestions to social workers and health visitors on how to include fathers that are wider in application than the field of child protection as narrowly construed. The book is extensively grounded in relevant theory, such as attachment theory.

Brigid Daniel is a Senior Lecturer at the Department of Applied Social Science and Social Work at Stirling University. Julia Taylor is Director of Postgraduate Studies at the School of Nursing and Midwifery Studies at the University of Dundee.

Golombok S (2000) *Parenting: What Really Counts?* Psychology Press, Hove.

Examining what is essential for a child's healthy psychological development, rather than advocating specific family structures, this study also examines children's attachments to their fathers and finds that, although fathers are children's preferred playmates, they need not necessarily be constrained to what might be said to be something of a stereotypical gender role, in that their caring can be just as beneficial for babies and older children as that of the mother.

Fathers Direct and National Family and Parenting Institute (2002) *How to Build New Dads. From Here to Paternity: supporting mothers by supporting fathers.* Fathers Direct and National Family and Parenting Institute, in association with the Home Office Family Policy Unit, London.

This publication, which is presented in a 16-page A4-size magazine format, targets health professionals working with new and expectant fathers. It makes the valuable point that with the introduction of paid paternity leave in 2003, health professionals will be likely to encounter more fathers around the time of the birth, particularly at home afterwards. It makes many good practice points about involving fathers, as well as background points about the value of doing so.

It founds the case for fathers largely on their supporter role – something which is perhaps open to question as tending to undermine the father's acquisition of his own skills and competences. It might also be argued that if health professionals only perceive fathers as supporters of women, they will continue to tend to overlook them (as at present) and will fail to implement those good proposals about engaging with fathers that are made by the booklet. *How to Build New Dads* also places a somewhat generalised emphasis on the value of group work with fathers.

Further reading

- Abrams R (2001) *Three Shoes, One Sock and No Hairbrush*. Cassell, London.
- Aiken C and George M (2000) *Surviving Postnatal Depression*. Jessica Kingsley Publishers, London.
- Birkett D (2000) Why little boys are not sex offenders. *Guardian*. **21 November**.
- Brunt S (2001) *Fathers in Child Protection: a brief look at the current situation*. National Society for the Prevention of Cruelty to Children, London.
- Buchanan A and Flouri E (2001) *Father Involvement and Outcomes in Adolescence and Adulthood*. Department of Social Policy and Social Work, Oxford University, Oxford.
- Burgess A (1998) *Fatherhood Reclaimed*. Vermillion, London.
- Burghes L, Clarke L and Cronin N (1997) *Fathers and Fatherhood in Britain*. Family Policy Studies Centre, London.
- Cameron C, Moss P and Owen C (1999) *Men in the Nursery: gender and caring work*. Sage, London.
- Clare A (2000) *On Men: masculinity in crisis*. Chatto & Windus, London.
- Daniel B and Taylor J (2001) *Engaging with Fathers: practice issues for health and social care*. Jessica Kingsley Publishers, London.
- Davidson N and Lloyd T (2001) *Boys' and Young Men's Health. Practice examples. Stage 1 interim report*. Working With Men for the Health Development Agency, London.
- Daycare Trust (2001) *Who Will Care? Recruiting the next generation of the childcare workforce*. Daycare Trust, London.
- Expert Maternity Group (1993) *Changing Childbirth. Part 1. Report of the Expert Maternity Group*. HMSO, London.
- Fathers Direct and National Childbirth Trust press release, *Government-funded Study of 'Blair Fathers' Demands Better Support for New Dads*, 11 September 2000.
- Ghate D, Shaw C and Hazel N (2000) *Fathers and Family Centres*. Joseph Rowntree Foundation, York.
- Gingerbread (2001) *Becoming Visible: focus on lone fathers*. Gingerbread, London.
- Golombok S (2000) *Parenting: what really counts?* Routledge, London.
- Hawkins AJ and Dollahite DC (1997) *Generative Fathering: beyond deficit perspectives*. Sage, Thousand Oaks, CA.
- Hazel N, Ghate D and Shaw C (2000) *Briefing Paper for Policy Makers and Service Providers: fathers and family support services*. Policy Research Bureau, London.
- Joseph Rowntree Foundation (2000) *A Man's Place in the Home: fathers and families in the UK*. Joseph Rowntree Foundation, York.
- Lavender T (1997) Can midwives respond to the needs of fathers? *Br J Midwifery*. **5**: 92–6.
- Lewis C (1986) *Becoming a Father*. Open University Press, Milton Keynes.
- Lewis C and Warin J (2001) *FatherFacts. Volume 1. Issue 1*. Fathers Direct, Newpin Fathers Support Centre, National Family and Parenting Institute and Working With Men, London.

- Lloyd T (2001) *What Works with Fathers?* Working With Men, London.
- Morrod D (2000) Brief encounters – picking up signals of relationship distress. *Pract Midwife.* **3**: 27–9.
- National Family and Parenting Institute (2001) *National Mapping of Family Support Services in England and Wales.* National Family and Parenting Institute, London.
- National Family and Parenting Institute (2002) *Reaching Parents: producing and delivering parent information resources.* National Family and Parenting Institute, London.
- National Society for the Prevention of Cruelty to Children (2000) *Child Maltreatment in the UK: a study of the prevalence of child abuse and neglect.* National Society for the Prevention of Cruelty to Children, London.
- *Becoming a Dad: what to expect*; nctpregnancyandbabycare.com, 15 February 2002.
- National Council of Voluntary Child Care Organisations (NCVCCO) and Kissman B (2001) *Are We Shutting Out Fathers? Conference Report.*
- O'Brien M and Shemilt I (2003) *Working Fathers, Earning and Caring.* Equal Opportunities Commission, London.
- Office for National Statistics (1999) *Labour Force Survey.* Office for National Statistics, London.
- Office for National Statistics (2001) *Social Focus on Men.* Office for National Statistics, London.
- OFSTED/HMI (2002) *Sex and Relationships. HMI 433. A Report from the Office of Her Majesty's Chief Inspector of Schools*; www.ofsted.gov.uk
- Phillips M (1999) A change in emphasis. *Sunday Times.* **30 May**.
- Prince's Trust (2001) *It's Like That: the views and hopes of disadvantaged young people.* Prince's Trust, London.
- Robertson A (1999) Get the fathers involved! The needs of men in pregnancy classes. *Pract Midwife.* **2**: 21–2.
- Royal College of Midwives (1994) *Men at Birth Survey.* Royal College of Midwives, London.
- Singh D and Newburn M (eds) (2000) *Access to Maternity Information and Support. The needs and experiences of women before and after birth.* National Childbirth Trust, London.
- Singh D and Newburn M (2000) *Becoming a Father.* National Childbirth Trust in association with Fathers Direct, London.
- Smith N (1999) Men in antenatal classes: teaching the whole birth thing. *Pract Midwife.* **2**: 23–6.
- Smith N (1999) Antenatal classes and the transition to fatherhood: a study of some fathers' views. *MIDIRS Midwifery Digest.* **9**: 463–8.
- Social Attitudes Survey (2001) Big rise in support for unmarried parents. *Guardian.* **26 November**.
- Speak S (1997) *Young Single Fathers. Participation in fatherhood – barriers and bridges.* Family Policy Studies Centre, London.
- UNICEF (2001) *A League Table of Child Deaths by Injury in Rich Nations. Innocenti Report Card.* UNICEF Innocenti Research Centre, Florence, pp. 20–1.
- Warin J, Solomon Y and Lewis C (1999) *Fathers, Work and Family Life.* Joseph Rowntree Foundation, York.
- Watson WJ, Watson L, Wetzel W *et al.* (1995) Transition to parenthood. What about fathers? *Can Fam Physician.* **41**: 807–12.

- White MB (1998) Men's concerns during pregnancy. Part 1. Re-evaluating the role of the expectant father. *Int J Childbirth Educ.* **13**: 14–17.
- Williams R (1999) *Going the Distance: fathers, health and health visiting*. University of Reading, Reading, in association with the Queen's Nursing Institute, London.
- Williamson H (1998) *Boys, Young Men and Fathers. Ministerial Seminar Report*. Home Office Voluntary and Community Unit, London.

News reports

- Australian MoT checks oil, plugs and exhaust – of men. *Electronic Telegraph*. 18 March 2001.
- Breastfeeding campaign targets men; *BBC News Online*, 15 May 2000.
- Fathers improve school results; *BBC News Online*, 28 February 2002.
- Fathers urged to quit smoking; *BBC News Online*, 9 June 2001.
- Internet site to make better men; *BBC News Online (Health)*, 14 November 2000.
- Men wanted in primary schools; *BBC News Online (Education)*, 22 April 2002.
- Men wreck smoke-free pregnancy; *BBC News Online*, 21 November 2001.
- Teen male suicides hit 'crisis level'; *BBC News Online (Health)*, 30 April 2001.
- Time to quit for the family; *BBC News Online (Business)*, 22 January 2002.
- Dobson R (2000) Children with father in family have a head start in life. *Sunday Times*. **21 May**.
- Dyer C (2001) Fathers picket judges over child access. *Guardian*. **30 October**.
- Hall S (2001) Crime linked to absent fathers. *Guardian*. **5 April**.
- Haughton E (2002) Men: your classroom needs you. *Independent*. **28 February**.
- Marin R (2000) At-home fathers step out to find they are not alone. *New York Times*. **2 January**.
- Park A *et al.* (2001) Big rise in support for unmarried parents (reporting on British Social Attitudes: the 18th report. Public policy, social ties). *Guardian*. **26 November**.
- Roberts J (2001) The tiny feet that trample romance. *Independent*. **30 July**.
- Smithers R (2002) Schools are short of male staff, admits minister. *Guardian*, **8 January**.

Men in Families Project

Rationale

The proposed programme recognises the importance of fathers in the lives of their children and the advantages of increasing both the motivation and skills of men in order to contribute positively to the well-being of their children.

The reasons for supporting fathers in their parenting role can be listed as follows.

1   In general, the role and impact of fathers is under-rated

Despite changes in recent years, much of the discussion around parenthood/childcare focuses on the role of mothers. The impact of fathers in building children's self-esteem, gender identity and school performance tends to be overlooked.

We have not taken sufficient pause as a society to count the social, economic and emotional costs of father absence, neglect and abuse. In resourcing and supporting parents, to focus on only half of the parenting equation is inequitable, shortsighted and ultimately not in our children's best interests.

2   Consequences for family life

Studies by Russell and others have consistently shown that women continue to perform the great majority of childcare tasks and household labour in general.

In terms of time, women perform approximately 90% of childcare tasks and 70% of all family work. Only 14% of fathers show a high level of participation in terms of time spent on family work.

Although public attitudes to gender roles in parenting and family life have changed, this change has not been matched by actual behaviour.

Greater equality in family life is associated with lower levels of family stress and higher levels of marital satisfaction for both mothers and fathers. This is especially so for fathers when they take more responsibility for the needs of their children.

3   Effects of fathers on children and child development

The perception of fathers as being uninvolved or unavailable to their children is all too common, and highly significant in terms of findings that the quality of fathering is related to the competence of both sons and daughters. Lack of attention from fathers has been related to low self-esteem, low self-control, diminished life-skills and less social competence among sons and daughters of primary school age.

As stated by Edgar, a new family policy should encourage new types of responsibility. First, *responsibility as fathers* means forming strong, loving and lasting bonds with their children. Secondly, *responsibility as partners* means changing their role in the household and learning to respect and treat women as individuals of equal worth.

4   The relationship between domestic violence and a lack of responsibility taken by men in family life

Anecdotal reports and some limited research indicate concern about the relationship between family violence and lack of participation by men in family tasks and nurturing roles.

Proposed target group

The target group for the proposed programme consists of all first-time fathers in Coffs Harbour on the Mid North Coast of New South Wales. Coffs Harbour is an area of high growth, with high numbers of young families, high indices of socio-economic disadvantage, high levels of domestic violence (much higher than State average increases in notifications of child abuse) and high levels of unemployment. The profile for young families in Coffs Harbour also includes risk factors common to many rural areas, such as lack of extended family and social support systems, and isolation and lack of appropriate services.

In 1997, statistics showed a high level of involvement of first-time fathers in antenatal classes in Coffs Harbour. Approximately 90% of first-time parents attended antenatal classes, and 95% of this figure attended classes as couples in evening programmes.

One of the most frequently cited difficulties with regard to the provision of services for men is the problem of access.

The proposed programme based on antenatal classes provides a unique opportunity to access men at a critical life stage that is characterised by a high level of motivation to contribute to the birth and development of their first child.

It is also noted by many service providers that a high percentage of couples maintain contact that is established through the antenatal classes, primarily because they have been through similar experiences at around the same time. It also appears that this continuing contact cuts across predicted associations based on education, employment and interests.

Experience and research increasingly support the benefits of early intervention programmes to support and develop parenting and relationship skills that contribute positively to all aspects of family life.

For many men, antenatal classes provide their first adult experience of groups. It is argued that these classes and the proposed 'follow-on' groups provide an opportunity to develop the ability of men to discuss a range of life issues and gain understanding and skills that are essential to their relationships with both their child and their partner.

The proposed programme provides a unique opportunity to support men in such areas as dealing with the transition to parenthood, understanding child development, development of the communication skills that are necessary in family relationships, and role negotiation and conflict resolution.

The development of mentors from the ongoing group will increase the number of positive role models and supports for men in their roles as parents and partners.

Programme details

The proposed programme will establish contact with new fathers through antenatal classes offered in Coffs Harbour. The participants will be invited to continue to meet after the birth, and the groups that are established will be developed and maintained by regular contact, information and continuing facilitation of group processes. The concept will build on the positive feelings and attitudes of prospective parents and, through a process of co-operative learning, will achieve the outcome of developing their roles both as parents and as partners.

It is also proposed that men will be selected from these groups to be trained as mentors for other men in their role as parents. This will achieve the outcome of increasing the number of positive role models who will play an active role in supporting fathers in all aspects of family life.

The programme will also act as an advocate for men in referrals to other services, and will address barriers that deter men from accessing help for issues relating to family life.

Goals

These can be summarised as follows:

1   to increase knowledge and adoption of appropriate parenting skills by new fathers in the Coffs Harbour District
2   to increase sharing of parenting roles and responsibilities within the targeted families
3   to develop appropriate anger management and conflict resolution skills in the target group
4   to increase men's knowledge of and access to supportive services in the community
5   to increase collaboration, public awareness, knowledge, skills and attitudes which support men in their roles both as parents and as partners.

Strategies

These can be summarised as follows:

1   to provide ongoing support to first-time fathers by continuing groups established in antenatal classes conducted in the targeted areas

- to increase the number of first-time fathers attending antenatal classes by:

  - giving publicity material to doctors, hospital staff and the general community

- to strengthen and expand groups that have been established in antenatal classes by developing group processes and extending an invitation to continue meeting after the birth by:

  - improving the skills and comfort of participants to enable them to benefit from group processes
  - promoting the benefits of accessing continuing support in their role both as parents and as partners

- to promote and develop positive parenting and relationship skills through the established support groups which are an extension of antenatal classes by:

  - providing information about child development
  - promoting the role of fathers and their importance for child development
  - promoting the sharing of parenting roles and responsibilities
  - developing the negotiation and communication skills that are critical for family life
  - facilitating the support role of ongoing groups

2   to develop selected fathers as mentors to provide support for men in their roles both as parents and as partners

- to encourage interested and suitable fathers to participate in the mentoring programme by:

  - discussing the mentoring programme in support groups
  - encouraging interested fathers to apply
  - developing an appropriate training programme in partnership with TAFE and Burnside.

Useful organisations

The following is a short list of organisations with expertise in working with new parents, men and fathers. The author does not guarantee that these organisations necessarily endorse the views expressed in this book.

The National Childbirth Trust (NCT)

This organisation provides information and support during pregnancy, childbirth and early parenthood, and has branches throughout the UK. The NCT wants all parents to have an experience of pregnancy, birth and early parenthood that enriches their lives and gives them confidence in being parents.

> The National Childbirth Trust (NCT)
> Alexandra House
> Oldham Terrace
> London W3 6NH
> Enquiry line: 0870 444 8707
> Breastfeeding line: 0870 444 8708 (information and support from breastfeeding counsellors who are available 7 days a week to talk about questions relating to baby feeding; fathers' support can be vital in helping partners to breastfeed)
> Website: www.nctpregnancyandbabycare.com
> Maternity sales:
>   Tel: 0870 112 1120
>   Website: www.nctms.co.uk

Fathers Direct

This charity, which was established in 1999, offers training and consultancy in working with fathers as well as a magazine for practitioners.

> Fathers Direct
> Herald House
> Lambs Passage
> Bunhill Row
> London EC1Y 8TQ
> Tel: 0207 920 9491
> Website: www.fathersdirect.com

Working With Men

This organisation, which was founded in 1988, provides resources, training and consultancy for projects and initiatives working with men and fathers.

Working With Men
320 Commercial Way
London SE15 1QN
Consultancy: 0207 732 9409
Resources: 0208 308 0709
Website: www.wwm-uk.freeuk.co.uk

Newpin Fathers' Project

This is the fathers' project of National NEWPIN, which works with fathers in mixed racial groups, young fathers' groups and black fathers' groups in an open and reflective way.

Newpin Fathers' Support Centre
The Amersham Centre
Inville Road
London SE17 2HY
Tel: 0207 740 8997
Email: fathers@nationalnewpin.freeserve.co.uk

Index

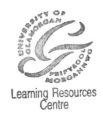